D0970671

SMALL BITES

Daily Inspirations

for

Weight Loss Surgery Patients

Other Books by Katie Jay

From the National Association for Weight Loss Surgery,
www.nawls.com

Dying to Change: My Really Heavy Life Story
How Weight Loss Surgery Gave Me Hope for Living

Coming in 2008...
When Even Surgery Isn't Enough:
What the Weight-Loss Doctors Haven't Told You
About How to Keep the Weight Off Permanently

Audio Products

Train to Maintain
Home Study Program

The WLS Mastery Series
Five experts talk about how to create WLS success

What people are saying about *Small Bites*

"The bariatric support community has a great friend in Katie Jay. Her ever-flowing words of encouragement and insight provide much needed and appreciated support for those who struggle each day to reach and maintain a healthy weight and lifestyle."

— Colleen Cook, President, Bariatric Support Centers International, www.bariatricsupportcenter.com

"It's about time a book like this was written. *Small Bites: Daily Inspirations for Weight Loss Surgery Patients* is a way of solving a very old problem for people who struggle with food and weight issues—it helps you change your unhealthy beliefs and build a stronger foundation for long-term success. Use this book as a tool to gain control of your eating and your life!"

— Dan Babbino, President, *WLS Lifestyles Magazine*, www.wlslifestyles.com

"*Small Bites: Daily Inspirations for Weight Loss Surgery Patients* is a day-to-day source of encouragement, wisdom, and practical information. I highly recommend it. Well done, Katie and Julia."

— Sally Myers, RD, CPT, Coauthor of *Caring for the Surgical Weight Loss Patient*

"What an insightful book! *Small Bites* gets to the heart of what it takes to make your weight loss surgery successful—a daily effort to change your old beliefs and behaviors, and to adopt a healthy lifestyle you can sustain."

— Jacqueline K. Smiertka, RN, Editor/Publisher, *Beyond Change* (www.beyondchange-obesity.com), and Coauthor of *Caring for the Surgical Weight Loss Patient*

from the National Association for
Weight Loss Surgery

SMALL BITES

Daily Inspirations

for

Weight Loss Surgery Patients

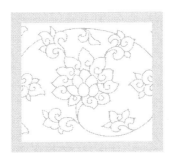

by Katie Jay and Julia A. F. Persing

Small Bites: Daily Inspirations for Weight Loss Surgery Patients by Katie Jay and Julia A. F. Persing

Published by Pink Sky Publishing, Inc. For information regarding distribution, please contact Pink Sky Publishing, Inc. at 1-877-PinkSky. ©2007 by Katie Jay. All rights reserved.

Publisher's Cataloging-In-Publication Data
(Prepared by The Donohue Group, Inc.)

Jay, Katie.
   Small bites : daily inspirations for weight loss surgery patients / by Katie Jay and Julia A. F. Persing.

   p. ; cm.

   Includes index.
   ISBN: 978-0-9772289-1-1

1. Gastric bypass--Patients--Miscellanea. 2. Gastric bypass--Miscellanea. 3. Affirmations. 4. Overweight persons--Conduct of life. I. Persing, Julia A. F. II. National Association for Weight Loss Surgery. III. Title. IV. Title: Daily inspirations for weight loss surgery patients V. Title: From the National Association for Weight Loss Surgery

BV4910.35 .J39 2007
242/.4   2007938478

To my beloved husband, Mike Jay, for saving my life.
To my son Barrett, who read and offered topics for this book.
And to Sarah, Charlie, Tyler, and Emily for loving me and
supporting me through a very difficult year.

— Katie Jay

To my husband David; children Treven, Barry, Camille and Kyle;
and my family who have been especially kind and patient with
me. To my friends for their prayers and support. A special thanks
to my mother who has always been there for me. And finally, to
God who inspired me and held my hand the whole time.

— Julia A. F. Persing

Introduction

As I was wheeled into the operating room for weight loss surgery (WLS), I knew down to my bones that my life was going to change forever. And I knew I would have to transform the physical, mental, and spiritual parts of me—not just my stomach—if I wanted to leave behind obesity for good.

But changing forever is hard.

WLS isn't magic. It didn't take away my old ideas—the ones that drive my choices and behavior. WLS didn't fix my belief system, self-esteem, or addiction to food. It was and is merely a physical tool for change.

I needed more than surgery. I needed to work on changing my heart and mind. That is what inspired me to write this book, along with my friend Julia Persing. I wanted a daily reader to help me change the way I think so that I could live a better life for the rest of my life, not just in the short term.

Small Bites: Daily Inspirations for Weight Loss Surgery Patients is a tool for mental and emotional change. In these pages you'll find topics to consider and actions to take so you can more easily create the psychological foundation for a life without obesity.

I encourage you to read a Small Bite each day for a full year, and to do the journaling exercises. You cannot help but be transformed if you truly give yourself over to this process.

If you'd like to discuss what you're reading in this book and how you're doing with the daily actions, join us at www.nawls.com, where you'll meet others who are taking the same journey.

We're all in this together.

Katie Jay

January

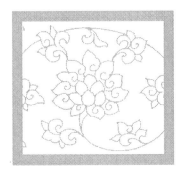

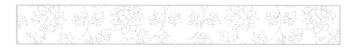

Set goals.

Resolutions are almost never successful. In fact, many of us make them knowing we will fail. Resolutions really are wishes, not commitments. This year, try something that is more likely to make your wishes come true: Set goals.

Goals are measurable and achievable. When you set a goal, do these three things: Write it down and post it where you will look at it often; list the steps you will take to achieve the goal; record your results.

Action for the day:

Pick a goal for this month. Write it down and post it on your bathroom mirror. List the steps you will take. Make a chart to record your progress.

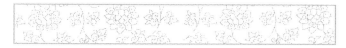

Be thankful.

Whether you admit it or not, you have many things to
be thankful for, including weight loss surgery, which has
given you the opportunity to overcome a devastating
health problem.

Take time to feel how thankful you are for each pound
lost and each clothing size, and how grateful you are to
walk without breathlessness.

Action for the day:

In your journal, begin a gratitude list to kick off this New
Year. Today, write down at least five things for which you
are grateful.

Learn the art of negotiation.

Living and working with non-WLS patients requires diplomacy. While you need a WLS-friendly environment at home and at work, others may feel strongly about bringing in unhealthy foods and beverages.

Negotiations can range from what to say during meals to what foods trigger you to overeat. The sooner you establish boundaries, the more comfortable everyone will be with your new lifestyle.

Action for the day:

In your journal, list three things friends, family, or coworkers do that add to your temptation and stress. Rehearse in your mind a negotiation process you can initiate. Begin that process today.

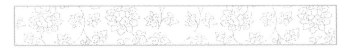

Transform gently.

With WLS, the changes in your body and your life are
dramatic. You may feel like you turned into someone else
entirely from the moment you underwent surgery. You
now have to eat differently, drink differently, and think
differently. You are controlled by schedules, checklists,
and your new plumbing.

Be gentle with yourself as you go through this metamorphosis.
Take your time. Give your body the chance to heal as
you adjust to your new look and your new way of eating
and living.

Action for the day:

Meditate on your vision of the transformed you. Then,
write down in your journal five things you want to accomplish
once you've reached your goal weight.

Rekindle your dreams.

Some WLS patients are very young and others have the
surgery later in life, yet at any time it is not too late to
become what you dream of becoming. Perhaps you
spend time in regret, thinking you should have had your
surgery sooner.

Focus on the present. You have more energy now than
you've had in years, and you can move more easily toward
your dreams.

Action for the day:

In your journal, describe something you want to
accomplish and make a list of the steps you need to take
to get there. Then, take one action that will move you
closer to your dream.

Eschew ignorance.

Learn all you can about WLS, even if you are well into your
recovery. The more you know about what is happening to
you and what could happen to you, the more comfortable
and successful you will be with the process. Read testimonials
from other patients. Discover what physical and emotional
challenges other people have experienced. Learn by
others' mistakes.

But remember, you will not experience every emotion, pain,
or problem others experience. And not all information sources
are reliable. Always check with your doctor before making
a change that could affect your health.

Action for the day:

Today, research an important WLS topic about which you
know little.

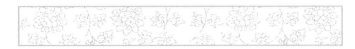

Accept success.

Accepting and embracing your new lifestyle will be the key to overcoming your obesity. To foster an attitude of acceptance, focus on where you are now, and what you can eat now. Rejoice in the quality of food you eat, not the quantity. Recognize that every day you follow your plan is a victory to celebrate.

The WLS journey is challenging, especially when you resist the lifestyle you know you must accept to succeed. Release the chains of doubt, defiance, desire, and regret. The world looks better when you see it from a fresh perspective—the perspective of acceptance.

Action for the day:

Whenever you feel resistance to your program, say to yourself, "I chose this new life. It is a gift I have given to myself and I'm going to make the most of it."

Get an accountability partner.

Your recovery is your responsibility, but don't go it alone. Find a partner to be accountable to, either someone in your support group or a friend. Having someone to call during moments of weakness can make a big difference. Your accountability partner can talk you down from eating the unhealthy food that is inches from your lips or encourage you to exercise.

Put your partner's phone number on your refrigerator, your pantry, and your phone. This person is an important part of your support system. You can be there for your partner, too, when he or she is in need.

Action for the day:

If you don't have an accountability partner, just ask someone. If they say no, ask someone else. If you do have an accountability partner, check in with him or her today.

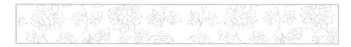

Value good nutrition.

You made the decision to make a dramatic change in your life. To get the most benefit from your WLS, think carefully about what you put into your body. With a smaller stomach, and/or shorter intestines, every bite of food must pack a nutritional punch.

Eat foods that will give you energy and the necessary building blocks for health. Every time you eat something, ask yourself, "Is this satisfying and making my body healthy?"

Action for the day:

Write down what you ate yesterday and what you are going to eat today. Are most of your food and supplement choices based on what your body needs or on what your head craves? Be honest with yourself.

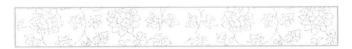

Make protein your nutritional foundation.

It's not always easy to get the protein you need, but it really is essential. Protein helps your body heal, helps keep your hair from falling out, stabilizes your blood sugar, and helps build muscle—among many other things.

If you are early out from surgery, you are probably using a protein supplement. Some people continue to use them. Protein supplements come in a wide variety of flavors. Sample as many as you need to until you find one you like. Don't give up on finding a supplement you can tolerate. The new you is not a quitter. The new you embraces the WLS lifestyle and accepts it for the tremendous freedom it brings.

Action for the day:

Count the number of protein grams you consume today. Are you on target? If not, make a better plan for tomorrow.

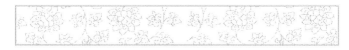

Identify safe, satisfying foods.

Probably one of the hardest things to get over is not being
able to eat everything you want. Yet, WLS is not a prison
sentence. It is a choice you made to reclaim your life—
an opportunity to enjoy life.

Eat foods that are good for you and that you really love.
Feed your hunger with flavor rather than volume. Concentrate
on eating slowly, savoring your food instead of gulping it.
Identify some satisfying, safe foods you can turn to when
you are struggling.

Action for the day:

In your journal make a list of "safe" foods you can eat that
are super satisfying.

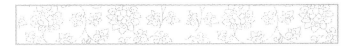

Develop a water strategy.

Do you find it difficult to drink enough water each day?
If so, it's time to think up a strategy to help you meet your
water-sipping goal.

Try filling a 32-ounce water bottle for on-the-go hydration.
Sip on it throughout the day. (You'll need to refill it once,
at some point.) Or, you can drink 8 ounces upon rising, 8
ounces mid-morning, 8 ounces 30 minutes before dinner, and
8 ounces at bedtime. You can keep bottled water in your car.
You can add lemon juice, cucumber slices, or mint leaves
to make your water more palatable. Think about what will
work for you. Don't let yourself off the hook. You can figure
this out.

Action for the day:

Make a plan for how you will drink 64 oz. of water today,
and follow it.

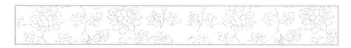

Make a schedule and follow it.

The reality is almost everyone who succeeds at losing weight and keeping it off uses some sort of schedule. A schedule helps keep you on track when the world is trying to interfere with your goals.

For example, following your schedule may help you manage your time, which in turn may give you more time to exercise. Not only can you achieve your WLS goals more easily when you use a schedule, you can have a fuller, more satisfying life.

Action for the day:

Make a schedule for today and see how well it works for you.

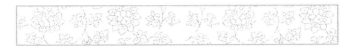

Take your new lifestyle seriously.

Your body is the only body you have to carry you through life. WLS requires you to learn to take care of it carefully.

Is taking vitamins part of your daily routine? Are you making healthy food choices to nourish your body? Are you getting enough physical activity? Accepting the obligations WLS places on you and taking them seriously will free you from your obesity.

Action for the day:

Today, show your resolve by being responsible for your health.

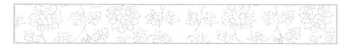

Surrender.

Some days you may wake up wishing you had the strength to meet the day's WLS demands. Chewing each bite is a challenge. You wish you could gulp a glass of water. You may feel you need additional motivation.

At these times of struggle, consider surrendering. Use a checklist or food plan as your definitive guide, and skip negotiating with yourself. Better days are ahead.

Action for the day:

Instead of rebelling to ease your disquiet, surrender to your WLS regimen today.

Accept life on life's terms.

Rather than think the whole world needs fixing, you can accept things today for what they are. You can choose to be disturbed that the world does not conform to your standards, or you can find joy in the people around you.

Accept who you are today—and accept others, no matter how imperfect they are.

Action for the day:

Today, look at the world through new eyes as a place to be appreciated, not changed.

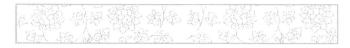

Trust your own judgment.

In most endeavors you undertake, there will be a line of people telling you how to do it. Some advice is great, but no matter how much you love, respect, or trust the people giving the advice, only you can judge if the advice is best for you.

When someone gives you advice you feel is wrong, you can always seek a second opinion. Respect other people's advice, thank them, and then make your own decision.

Action for the day:

Concentrate today on being your own person, while keeping an open mind.

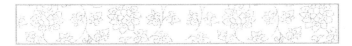

Communicate with your family.

Sometimes it's depressing to be reminded of the old adage:
You can pick your friends, but not your family. You may need
to teach your family to contribute to your long-term WLS
success if they don't warm up to the idea naturally. Some
family members may not understand the level of change
required in your life. While others may think your surgery
was too extreme.

Try to be patient and gentle with them. Explain your
WLS lifestyle to them as clearly as you can, and make your
two-way communication ongoing.

Action for the day:

Today, practice communicating your needs to your family,
while also listening to their concerns.

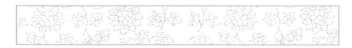

Show compassion for others.

The major changes brought about by your WLS may lead
you to focus inward. It's easy to become self-absorbed during
this physical and mental transformation.

Remember the people around you. As a WLS patient, it is
important to be kind to yourself, but as you extend kindness
to others you'll create harmony with everyone you encounter.

Action for the day:

Today, especially if you've been self-absorbed lately,
spend some time and energy thinking about others' needs
and desires.

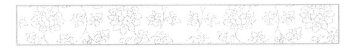

Measure your progress.

Plateaus are common on a WLS journey, but don't despair.
Often you are losing inches even when the scale is not
inching down.

That is why you are encouraged to take your measurements.
Keeping track of your measurements is a wonderful way to
chart your progress. Even after you reach goal, you can see
how your exercise regimen is changing your body.

Action for the day:

No matter where you are on your journey, take your
measurements today. Then wait a month and measure again.

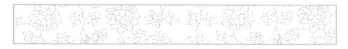

Let go to move forward.

When you hold on to resentment you cause yourself stress.
You also take your focus away from your goals. Your
grudges can distract you without even solving a past wrong.

You may be holding a grudge against a person who is not
even aware that you are hurt. You could be wasting valuable
energy and mental power on an issue that has no bearing
on your future. It's time to seek understanding, forgive,
and move on.

Action for the day:

In your journal, write about any lingering resentments.
Resolve to do what is necessary for you to forgive and move
on. Seek help if you need it.

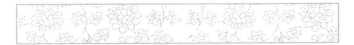

Create a supportive community to meet your needs.

Many WLS patients long for support, but live in an area that lacks resources. If you are in that situation, consider starting your own support group.

Another great reason to start a support group is if your own group is toxic. In other words, if your group is not solution focused, with lots of people working hard to succeed, you might consider starting a group of your own that will meet your needs.

Action for the day:

If you don't have a healthy group available to you, research how to create a community of caring and supportive people to help you reach your goals.

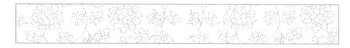

Help your family and friends change with you.

You may be right when you think that none of your family or friends understand your WLS experience. These people are not you. The best strategy for peace is to love and teach one another. You have made a choice. Rather than get angry or resentful because a family member or friend comes in eating a sugary food with a tempting aroma, teach them how to support your goal of long-term WLS success.

Realize your family and friends must learn how to fulfill their needs while supporting you. Finding the right balance will take time and communication. Just keep at it.

Action for the day:

Forgive your family members and your friends, as you teach them how to support you.

Fill your WLS toolbox.

A carpenter uses tools to carve beautiful designs. Likewise, you will use tools to shape your long-term WLS success. Collect them.

Learn new skills, try new strategies, and gather information. All these things will give you tools for your toolbox. Your consistent efforts to fill your toolbox, and then to use the tools, will help you achieve your goals.

Action for the day:

Add to your WLS toolbox by learning something new today.

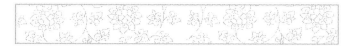

Let go of procrastination.

Putting off the things you need to do—like taking vitamins, replacing protein supplements when they run out, or starting an exercise program—is a luxury you can't afford after WLS.

Procrastination often is fear of imperfection or fear of failure. But no one said you have to be perfect on your WLS journey. You just need to keep moving forward.

Action for the day:

Make a list of the things you must do for your health today and check them off as you accomplish them. If you feel resistant, call someone who supports you and talk about it.

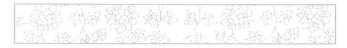

Make peace with your limitations.

Because WLS is a life-time journey, your post-op life will include both extreme highs and extreme lows, and there will be times when making a healthy choice is very hard.

You can look back and review how you've handled challenging situations in the past to get clues about how you will handle them in the future. Identify your weak areas, so that you will know what kind of support you'll need. It's okay to have limitations. Just make a plan for how you will handle them.

Action for the day:

In your journal, explore how you've handled extreme times in the past. Make a list of your areas of vulnerability. Think about how you can get support so that your limitations don't become major setbacks.

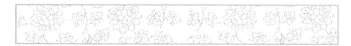

Give your gifts to the world.

Everyone has gifts to share. You may think you are not
blessed with gifts, that you have no special talent, but that
is not true. What do you enjoy doing? What kinds of things
are you good at? Have you helped someone? What do people
turn to you for? The answers to these questions will reveal
your gifts.

A gift does not need to be a spectacular talent like playing
classical piano at the age of three; it could simply be the
ability to show compassion. Your gifts are meant to be shared
with the world, to make it a better place.

Action for the day:

Make a list of your talents, gifts, and strengths. How can
you help a neighbor? Your community? Take an action today
that utilizes one of your gifts.

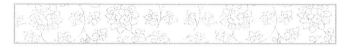

Love your new face.

As you lose weight, your rounded face changes. The double chins fall away and your baby face begins to mature into an adult face, with perhaps a bit of sagging skin. The person you see in the mirror is unfamiliar to you, but he or she is the mature and vibrant you. It may take you awhile to see your new face and body as they really are, rather than the distorted interpretation you may see now.

You will see yourself more accurately the further out from surgery you get. Give yourself a couple of years. It takes time.

Action for the day:

What you say to yourself about yourself will affect how you think and feel. Write down a positive affirmation about how you look and say it to yourself every morning as you look in the mirror. Notice how this changes your thoughts and feelings about yourself.

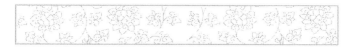

Cultivate an independent attitude.

What does it mean to be independent? It means freedom from the control and influence of others. To be truly successful with WLS you need to detach yourself from the influences of society and depend on your own judgment.

Being independent of action does not mean you need to isolate yourself from society. But, when others around you are indulging, you need to develop the ability to make a different choice. It is not shameful to say no to food. You can determine what is good for you in a situation and be confident in your choices. Participating in society, yet ultimately making your own decisions, is true freedom.

Action for the day:

True friends will respect your independence. Make a choice today that honors your WLS lifestyle.

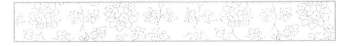

Embrace your Shar-pei look.

As the pounds melt away, your skin may get a bit droopy.
Just like the Shar-pei dogs with the many folds of sagging
skin, you too will be lovable, soft, and healthy. Your loose
skin may tighten up in time, or you may choose to have it
surgically helped along.

Yet, is it not better to have the sagging skin, proud scars of
your battle, than to be sick? Would you trade that skin for
diabetes, sleep apnea, high blood pressure, heart disease,
cancer risks, breathlessness, and immobility? Resolve not to
be distressed by loose skin. It is only on the outside. Inside
you are healthier, happier, and still you. Acknowledge the
sagging skin as a positive change, for it is an indicator that
WLS is working for you. You are fulfilling your commitment
to yourself.

Action for the day:

Make a list of the things you can do now, that you could not
do before you had weight loss surgery.

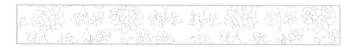

Spend anger wisely.

One of the hardest emotions to master is anger. Handled
unwisely, it can be costly. Whether your anger is justified or
not, wallowing in it is a luxury you cannot afford. Anger can
lead to self-destructive behavior, which can undermine your
WLS success. When you feel anger, allow yourself a private
moment to think things through. What will be the consequences? Will you alienate a friend who has been supportive?
Will you affect your position at work? Will your anger cause
you to overeat?

If thinking through consequences does not dissipate your
anger, then you can remove yourself from the situation
completely and cool off. Try again to resolve your issue when
your emotions have settled down.

Action for the day:

Think about how you deal with anger. Does your anger hurt
you or others? Plan a strategy to implement when your anger
rises. Get help if you need it.

February

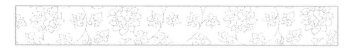

Move forward with optimism.

Practice an optimistic outlook—a hopeful and eager view—
to multiply your chances of success. Optimism puts into
play a powerful force on your behalf. Even when life is hard,
know that nothing lasts forever. As you have heard before,
"This, too, shall pass."

It's easy to get discouraged when you have had a lot of
practice being discouraged. But, now it's time to practice
optimism.

Action for the day:

Pay attention to your thoughts today. When you have a
negative thought, immediately replace it with an optimistic
thought. Optimism can be learned.

Laugh to lighten your load.

Laughing releases endorphins, those chemicals in your brain that make you feel good. Even if you don't feel like laughing, the act of laughing will make you feel better. If your goal is to feel better—healthier, happier, more relaxed—then adding laughter to your day makes sense.

Exercising your mental happiness is as important as exercising your body. Think of it as internal aerobics. Strengthen your sense of humor so that when strain after strain is beating you down, you can fight back with laughter.

Action for the day:

No matter how silly you feel, set a timer and laugh for three minutes today—whether you feel happy or not. See what happens!

Dare to experiment.

Life is brimming with experiences to be lived—and now
you are physically able to experiment. After surgery, you
certainly tried new foods; but now it is time to experiment
in other areas.

Try on a new style of clothes. Experiment with square dancing
or a spirited aerobics class. How about learning a musical
instrument now that you're breathing easier? Join a book club
or a Bible study without fear of breaking a chair. Whatever
looks interesting to you, try it. Imagine life is a buffet, and it's
your mission to sample the many treats it has to offer.

Action for the day:

What new experience do you want to have? Take action
toward that goal today.

Persevere.

Some days you wake up feeling tired or distracted. You just don't have the time or energy to follow your WLS regimen at that moment. So, you skip breakfast, or eat that slice of cold pizza that you righteously avoided the night before. Days of discouragement shouldn't surprise you. They are reminders that food will always be complicated—either a comfort or a distraction.

The key to real change is perseverance. When you take a misstep, for whatever reason, know that you will continue to persevere in your WLS recovery. You will start over at the next meal—you will overcome the temptation next time. That is how you'll succeed. Being perfect just isn't going to happen. So persevere.

Action for the day:

No matter where you are in your recovery, today you will persevere. Start over every time you stray from your plan. Start over as often as necessary.

Believe you can.

Believing the improbable can happen is the first step to making it happen. People can get mired down in believing that their current way of life will never change. They imagine they will be stuck in their rut forever and they stop trying.

But, the truth is change rewards you when you work for it. You changed your life and your health with surgery. Now you can consider changing other parts of your life. You might want to make new friends, to stop obsessing about food, or to make a career change. Visualize where you want to be, and then work toward that goal. You'll be amazed at how the world opens before you.

Action for the day:

Find a quiet, private space where you can relax and breathe for five minutes. During your quiet time, visualize your life as you want it to be. Imagine as many details as you can. What are you wearing? Who is with you? What excites you? Allow yourself to feel the pleasure of that new life. Describe it in your journal.

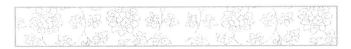

Find the answers inside you.

Let's face it, many of us had WLS because we were desperate to be healthy and productive. We wanted to chase our kids, grocery shop without the "go cart," or sit comfortably in a theatre seat.

Now that you are smaller, you have different needs. You feel restless, but you don't know what you want. Know that the solution resides inside of you. Your small inner voice knows what you need to do differently, knows what you are avoiding, knows what you desire. Life-transforming WLS recovery requires introspection. So, look inside. And, if you need therapy, get it. No excuses! If you have to get out of your comfort zone, do it. Start the journey within.

Action for the day:

Today, resolve to know the inside of you as well as you know the outside. As you heal your body, resolve to heal your soul, in part, by understanding your inner self.

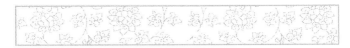

Use exercise as a tool.

Some people love to exercise. As WLS returns their bodies
to a healthier, more able form, they embrace exercise with
a renewed vigor. Other people do not love exercise, but
know that it is considered an essential part of an effective
WLS program.

If you are not fond of exercise, it's time to work on changing
your mind about it. Exercise is your lifeline. It will make your
weight loss and maintenance much, much easier. To make it
more palatable, try something entertaining. You can put on
music and dance, ride a bike, buy an exercise video that
appeals to you, garden, listen to a book on tape while you
walk, or find a friend to walk with. Exercise does not have to
be torture.

Action for the day:

Move your body today in some new way. Also, plan what
exercise you'll do for the rest of the week and put it on your
calendar. If you worry you may not exercise at a planned
time, schedule something with a friend to motivate you.

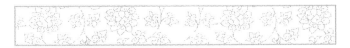

Listen to your body and trust yourself.

While somewhat rare, WLS puts people at risk for complications. If anything concerns you, ignoring it and hoping it gets
better may turn something simple into something serious.
Your surgeon, or your primary care physician, is often the best
judge if something is wrong.

But if you do not agree with your doctor, don't be shy about
getting a second opinion. You are responsible for your health.
If the solution the surgeon offers does not work, call back.
If you are in serious distress don't be shy about going to the
emergency room. The new you takes care of him or herself
and tackles health problems head on. Learn about the
common complications that can happen after WLS and avoid
unnecessary suffering.

Action for the day:

If you have medical questions or concerns, call your surgeon
or primary care physician today and get them addressed.
You deserve to be healthy and comfortable.

Reassure loved ones.

The special people in your life will go through a flood of emotions as you transform before their eyes. Your spouse, family, or friends may feel insecure as you approach your goal weight. When you were large, they may never have feared losing your love and attention. Now that you are thinner, and especially if you get thinner than they are, they may fear that you will not want to spend time with them or that you will leave.

Be reassuring. If your loved ones feel threatened by your new body, they may try to sabotage your efforts. Help them realize that you still want to be in a relationship with them, and that you are willing to work things out.

Action for the day:

Look a loved one in the eye today and tell him or her you love them. Thank them for supporting you. And offer reassurance.

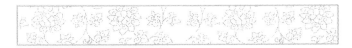

Take responsibility.

The quality of your life is the result of your reactions to life. When you are faced with a challenge, be it a health issue or something else, the final outcome is either positive or negative based on how you react.

Taking responsibility for your obesity means reacting positively to the demands of your surgery—rather than feeling sorry for yourself or feeling rebellious. Taking responsibility means you control the outcome of your surgery.

Action for the day:

In your journal, write down three things in your life that are bothering you—things that make you feel like a victim. Next to each item, write down a realistic response you could have that would improve the situation—and your perception of yourself.

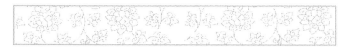

Pain is a message; listen to it.

Listening to your pain when everything around you says ignoring it shows strength, is really strength. Pain is a message that indicates something is wrong. Physical pain may mean you are working too hard, or it may mean you're sick. Emotional pain is also an indicator that something is not right. This pain is very real and can be quite damaging, too. Many people overeat when they have emotional pain.

If you ignore your pain and do not attend to it, your pain is likely to grow. If you need to, seek help. Even if you think you are being silly or weak, remind yourself you are not. You were not created to live in isolation. Getting help when you need it makes a world of difference.

Action for the day:

Today, if you are suffering with pain of any kind, spend some time considering what will soothe it. Connect with at least one gentle person today to discuss your discomfort.

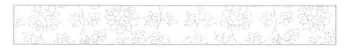

Step out of your comfort zone.

There comes a time when what you are doing stops working well. Then, it's time to try something new—whether you need to change your exercise routine, avoid a food that has become a trigger for overeating, or ask for support.

Unfortunately, most people get very comfortable with their routines and habits. Too comfortable. Maybe the thought of changing makes you angry or afraid. Some change is healthy. It helps you grow (or shrink as the case may be). You may need to get a personal trainer to help you learn how to boost your metabolism, or see a nutritionist about adjusting your menu. As the saying goes, feel your fear and make the change anyway. Long-term WLS success requires you to step out of your comfort zone.

Action for the day:

When the tried and true stops working, it's time to try something new. Be honest with yourself. What do you need to change? Get out of your comfort zone and try something new today.

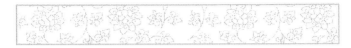

Appreciate imperfection.

Some of the most precious gems in the world have flaws that do not diminish their worth. When a diamond is a deep yellow or brown, it is considered more valuable. So, what you might assume is a serious flaw is really a great strength.

Do you judge yourself by impossible standards? Do you berate yourself for lack of perfection? Your flaws make you unique and precious. Your sensitivity means you are compassionate. Not looking perfect makes you approachable. Surviving pain brings others hope. You are not a worthless rock; you are a precious gem.

Action for the day:

Think of three people you admire. In your journal, describe their flaws. How do their flaws make them unique and precious? What flaws might people appreciate in you?

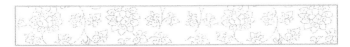

Drop some rocks.

We live in a busy world. Often success is measured by how much we do, how busy we are, and how heavy the load is that we carry. Imagine that your job in life is to swim across a fast-moving river carrying a bag of rocks. People often fill their bags with too many rocks, including rocks that don't belong to them.

Are you carrying other people's rocks? Are you doing all the work for the team at your job? Are you volunteering again because no other parent stepped up? Carrying more rocks than you need is risky. Carrying your rocks and everyone else's will sabotage your WLS recovery.

Action for the day:

In your journal today, make a list of the rocks in your bag— your various responsibilities. Drop at least one of the rocks that doesn't belong to you.

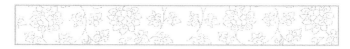

Resolve to stop "escape eating."

Many WLS patients have overeaten for years, in part to escape certain feelings. You might have eaten to escape feelings of anxiety, depression, sadness, boredom, or being overwhelmed. After WLS, many people continue to engage in escape eating.

It's time to ask yourself, "How well is escape eating working for me?" Is it moving you toward your long-term WLS goals? Is it a nagging problem that you're managing, but that could get out of control over time? Changing this pattern means identifying your feelings and choosing a new response to those feelings. You do have a choice.

Action for the day:

Record what you eat for three days. Beside each entry, write down how you were feeling when you ate. Were you hungry? Were you lonely, angry, or tired? This activity will help you identify and curb your emotional triggers.

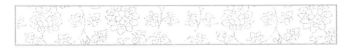

Focus on today.

Time spent thinking about regrets and past hurts is time
wasted. You cannot go back and make different decisions,
better choices. You cannot change the past hurts others have
caused you. By dwelling on them today, you are hurting
yourself all over again.

You only have today. Today is an opportunity to take actions
and make choices that will cause you no regrets tomorrow.
Today, if you feel wronged, you can express your feelings in
the moment, forgive, and move on. Today is the day to do
well the things you can do, and let go of the rest. Your
yesterdays are only experiences you will use to help you
make healthier choices today.

Action for the day:

Whenever a regret comes up, or a resentment, acknowledge
it and then turn your thoughts to the present. What can you
do to make it a healthy and peaceful day today?

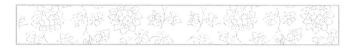

Own your truth.

The truth may be you are not drinking all your water, or you may be skipping your morning protein supplement because you don't want to take the time. The truth may be you don't take your multi-vitamin because you don't like it. You may be too tired and want to give up, so you tell yourself you're just backing off a little. You let yourself off the hook and decide you'll recommit next week when you are not so tired (or busy, or sad, or stressed).

These choices are a red flag that you are slipping away from your commitment to overcome obesity. If you are finding more and more that you don't want to do the things that make and keep you healthy, you should consider getting back to basics and seeking help. Waiting will only make your situation worse.

Action for the day:

Is there something you know you need to be doing that you have been avoiding? Make a plan to get yourself back on track. Own your truth today.

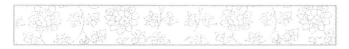

Create a habit of success.

Part of being successful with WLS is learning to make success, in general, a habit. Set a goal (but not a weight goal) that you will achieve each month, no matter what. Maybe you will paint a room this month. Next month, you will clean the attic. The following month you might write letters to several old friends—whatever you can think up. Just have a monthly goal and complete it no matter what it takes.

Building a list of accomplishments will put you into a positive frame of mind. If you still have a few pounds to lose, don't fret. You have proven to yourself you get done what you make up your mind to do. This can-do mindset is very powerful as it applies to EVERY goal you set.

Action for the day:

In your journal, make a list of potential, non-weight-related goals you can strive for in the coming months. Pick a manageable one to accomplish before the end of this month. Keep it realistic, and do it no matter what.

Nurture happiness.

Do you want something so badly you've become obsessed?
Do you desire some object or goal so much that you've
forgotten to enjoy the wonderful things you already have?
What if, when you finally obtain that object or reach that
goal, it is not all that you imagined?

It's time to develop the belief that you already have all you
need to be happy. You are blessed with many things you
refuse to see. You only focus on what you do not possess.
Until you are satisfied with what you have, and with who
you are, achieving goals will bring only empty victory.
Happiness begins now, not someday.

Action for the day:

What goals are you obsessing about, thinking you'll be
happy only when you achieve them? How can you find more
happiness in today? Do something today that nurtures
happiness in the present moment.

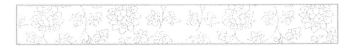

Keep it green.

There are two good reasons to keep memories of your former self fresh and green. The first reason is so that you do not repeat past mistakes. Your new self does not want to give up and go back to past behavior. The other reason to keep your past fresh in your mind is for encouragement when you are feeling you don't look any different or you aren't where you want to be.

When you look back, you can see the difference. Remember how ill you were and how much better you feel now. Although you may want to forget the pain of your obesity, the remembrance of your old self is a valuable tool for success.

Action for the day:

Meditate on how you used to live your life before surgery. Close your eyes and imagine how you used to climb the stairs or how it used to feel squeezing into a chair or booth. Keep your memory green.

Believe you can overcome obesity.

To succeed at anything you first must have the belief that it can be accomplished. Even though it is imperfect, WLS can be a phenomenal tool in your battle with obesity. But, you must believe and accept that YOU can make this tool work for you. You can do this.

When you had your surgery, you looked inside yourself and found the strength to mold your own destiny. You have turned yourself around in what seemed a dark tunnel of impossibility, and you have faced the light. Surgery is the beginning of believing that you will lose weight and keep it off. It is up to you to keep this faith alive. Feed your faith as you find a healthier way to feed your body.

Action for the day:

Today, write a letter to yourself, assuring yourself you are in control. This is just one way to nurture the new faith that is taking root in your life. You have the ability to succeed with WLS.

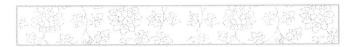

Respect your triggers.

Maybe you let your son buy chips at the store yesterday.
Or you have eaten at restaurants more often lately. Did you
offer to bake something to bring to a party—something you
know will trigger food cravings in you? Once on the road to
recovery, you may feel that you can handle more temptations.
Sometimes you can. And sometimes allowing your food
triggers to creep back into your life is a recipe for disaster.

Your triggers are a part of you and must be acknowledged
and respected. Obesity is a deadly disease, and you have it,
whether you are thin or heavy. It's time to gently tell yourself,
"No." There are some foods you just can't be around safely.
Staying away from a trigger food is a one-day-at-a-time
challenge. But you can do it.

Action for the day:

Make an honest list of your trigger foods. Are any of them in
your house? Ask a friend to help you get rid of them now. It
will never get any easier. Not even after you've gained 10
pounds. So do it now.

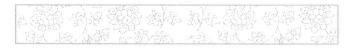

Explore your healthy options.

The world is full of wonderful foods that taste good and are good for you. Thankfully, the produce area of the grocery store is an international delight of exotic fruits and vegetables. Sweet cravings can be fulfilled by small servings of juicy melons, decadent star fruits, and plump berries. When you want something salty, tomatoes and olives do the trick. What about needing to satisfy that urge just to crunch? Then chew on some celery, colorful peppers, raw asparagus, or cucumbers. When you crave a spice from an old favorite food, it can easily be incorporated into your healthy diet. For example, garlic, onion powder, paprika, and oregano are popular flavors for fried foods, but these can also be incorporated into meat mixes or added to the water in which you cook whole grains.

When you step outside of your eating comfort zone, the rewards can be great and healthy. Sampling a variety of foods will prove invaluable to your new way of eating.

Action for the day:

Be thankful you have so many healthy food options. Try a new, healthy food today.

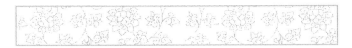

Make gratitude your new point of view.

Grateful recognition of the sacrifices people around you
have made will increase your own sense of personal power
and wellness. When you show gratitude for gifts from
others, whether they be material or emotional gifts, you
are rewarded.

People will endure many hardships if they know that their
efforts are appreciated and recognized. Showing gratitude is a
way of encouraging others to support you. And what if the
gifts are sometimes well-meaning flops? You know all too well
what it is like to be judged. You can rise above judgment and
show your appreciation for what others have given—even if
their gifts are not perfect.

Action for the day:

Show appreciation to one of your supporters today. Secretly
do something nice for one of them. (And remember, you
don't have to be perfect, either!)

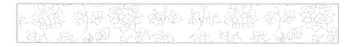

Redefine your idea of beauty.

True beauty comes from within. Even though what's on the outside is important to most of us, remember that a person who is pleasing to the eye, if they have an ugly soul, will not find peace. Think of the most beautiful person you know. What qualities does that person possess? From that list you will notice not all their beauty is on the outside. Now think about what is wrong with their appearance.

Even with flaws people are beautiful. You are, too. No matter what your body ends up looking like when you reach your goal, you are still beautiful. (Yep, even with the sagging skin!) Your beauty radiates from within. Your beauty is not only skin deep.

Action for the day:

To cultivate the beauty within you, in your journal list five things you have done in your life that show your inner beauty. Meditate on why and how these things reflect your inner beauty.

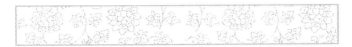

Act first.

If you wait to be inspired before you move into action, you will not get much accomplished. Seldom does anything worthwhile happen if you wait for inspiration. Inspiration is born of action.

To achieve, you must be willing to act first and follow each small step to your goal. Even a small step is progress. Progress toward a goal is often all the inspiration you need to keep you going. And before you know it, you've reached your goal.

Action for the day:

Take a small action toward a goal today, whether you want to or not.

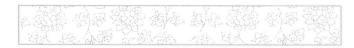

Be a force for change—not a victim.

Are you frustrated with people and situations you want to change? Longing for the world to change to make things easier for you won't help. The only way change occurs is if you take responsibility and make the effort (and have the courage) to do something different—despite what others may think or say.

To bring about the changes that support your WLS lifestyle, you can resolve to treat gatherings as opportunities to have fun and be social, rather than to eat. You can serve healthy foods when eating is a necessary part of an event. You can heighten awareness of healthy foods and portion sizes, and you can change your own environment to suit your needs. You can be a gentle and confident example who inspires others.

Action for the day:

Resolve to be a force for change in the world. Make the choice to stick up for your own needs today.

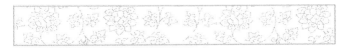

Find new ways to nurture yourself.

Sometimes people use food as a way of nurturing themselves.
Food is such a comfort when you are feeling down. It is a
great companion when you are celebrating alone. It brings
true pleasure, both in the anticipation of eating it and with
the first bite. Yes, food is nurturing.

After WLS, it's still okay to enjoy food. In fact, eating the
highest quality of food you can afford, and preparing it well,
helps you to feel satisfied with your new life. However, a
healthy approach to dining dictates you eat only when you
really need to. When you want to eat, but know you're not
hungry, identify the feelings behind your desire to eat. Are
you in need of nurturing? If so, choose an alternative to food.
You'll get used to responding differently to your nurturing
need. Give it time.

Action for the day:

Make a list in your journal of things that feel nurturing to
you other than eating. The next time you feel the need to be
nurtured, try something from this list.

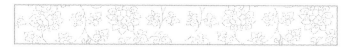

Fulfill your role.

Everyone has their perfect part to play in the unfolding of
the universe. You have a niche to fill, a place you are
destined to be, a job you are meant to do. Many people feel
a longing for purpose, but have not yet figured out just
what that purpose is. What is your role in this world? Maybe
you have always known, or maybe you are still searching.

Sometimes people don't fill their niche because they are
afraid. Maybe when you were obese you were physically
unable to follow your purpose. If you meditate on what really
excites you, and on your skills and abilities, you will find your
purpose. Maybe the answer is right in front of you waiting to
be recognized. If you know what your purpose is, but are
afraid, talk about that with someone you trust and admire.

Action for the day:

In your journal, create a mission statement for your life.
If you don't know what that means or how to do it, search
on the Internet to find out.

March

Perform a miracle.

Maybe you don't feel like you have the energy or ability to work a miracle, but you do. Sometimes, one small change can bring about great things. And you can make one small change. Maybe you can get up 30 minutes earlier and do a yoga video. Or you can fill out a WLS food plan for the day. Just one small thing.

After surgery, one WLS patient began walking 5 minutes a day. Every week she added 5 minutes to her walk. Now, a year later, she walks 3 miles a day and it feels effortless. Three miles is a miracle, when compared with the painful half block she could hobble before WLS. But the miracle doesn't stop there. She joined a hiking club and met a wonderful man. They recently married and are expecting their first child. That little baby is yet another miracle.

Action for the day:

Are you ready to work miracles? Start today by making one small change. If you feel overwhelmed, make it one tiny change. But do it and don't give up on it. See what miracles your small change leads to over time!

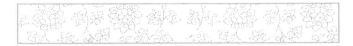

Recognize your worthiness.

There are those of us who think we are not worthy of success. We cannot accept prosperity. But how happy are you when you see an underdog succeed? How genuine is your praise of other people who have struggled to reach a goal?

The joy you feel for another person is the same as the joy someone feels for you when you reach your goals. Accept praise with joy and gratitude. Don't say, "It was nothing." You are worthy of praise and you have earned it. You only diminish the joy of others when you dismiss their praise of you. The rewards of your work are not just the numbers on the scale or your pants size, but also the respect and recognition you get from friends and family.

Action for the day:

Allow people to share their joy for you. It is a gift you can give them that will lift you up, too.

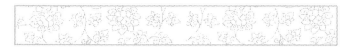

Be here in this moment.

Sometimes the best way to get through the day is to choose
to be present and enjoy the moment. Dwelling on things you
cannot change or allowing yourself to be consumed by what
might happen tomorrow takes away the joy of the moment.

Children have perfected the skill of living in the moment.
For them, only the slide exists and the sheer joy they embody
as they zip down it. You can live by their example. Focus
on the moment as it is happening. Laugh with your loved
ones. Scratch your cat behind the ears and sense its pleasure.
Rejoice in the success of a friend. Experience the joys of
today as if today were the only day you have.

Action for the day:

Be present and find joy in each moment today.

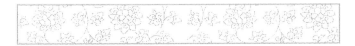

See yourself in a positive light.

Shar-pei dogs have luxurious folds of soft skin. They're really cute. After WLS, people develop folds of skin as they lose weight, but most don't find those folds cute. To tolerate the folds from an emotional standpoint, it's important to look at things from a kinder perspective.

Use positive affirmations and self talk to help you accept (and even admire) your new appearance. After all, you're not morbidly obese anymore. Your health is improved. And you have energy and abilities that used to be out of reach. The positive benefits beat the negatives by far—if you look at your situation with nonjudgmental eyes.

Action for the day:

When you look in the mirror today, smile and pick out something you like about the way you look. Don't leave the mirror until you think and feel something positive.

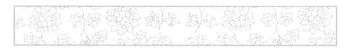

Identify and avoid your trigger foods.

Do you tell yourself one bite won't hurt? Sometimes one bite
is just fine, but sometimes it isn't. You are the only person
who can make that determination. The key is to find the
balance between deprivation and indulgence. If you take a
bite or two, walk away, and don't think about the food again
for days, you're probably okay.

If, however, you have a bite and spend all of your free time
thinking about the next bite, it's probably a trigger food that
you should consider avoiding. If you don't avoid the trigger
foods, one bite leads to another and another. Is it worth it?
The new you says, "No, I want to live a full, healthy life.
I will not go back to the old pain and suffering. I have a
choice today."

Action for the day:

Review your list of trigger foods in your journal. Try to avoid
your trigger foods just for today.

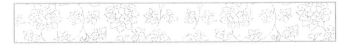

Feel your fear and do it anyway.

Sometimes your perception of how a situation will unfold
keeps you from attempting the activity. You imagine how
uncomfortable it's going to be and you don't want to take
the risk. Yet, sometimes you just need to take a deep breath
and accept the invitation to try. Most of the time it's not as
bad as you think. You may find you actually have a good
time, make a few new friends, and learn some new things.
Accepting the challenge enables you to rise to the occasion
and profit from the experience.

Even when the situation does not work out, you have learned
something, and you have established a new pattern of risk
taking. The new you will not let fear be the only reason for
not taking a risk. You are becoming more capable every day,
and you are living your life accordingly.

Action for the day:

Think about what holds you back from fully participating in
life. Give yourself permission to take the risk to be a part of
something exciting today.

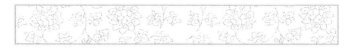

Stand up for your needs.

When it's time for you to do something for yourself, like exercise or take your vitamins, it's okay to do it—even if others want you to do something for them instead. Resist the temptation to put off until later what you know is necessary now. Except in very rare circumstances, another's needs should not completely supersede your own. You may be trying not to offend someone or trying not to bring attention to yourself, but if your ultimate goal is to live a healthy life, consider reexamining your values.

Your needs and goals have changed. When you decide to grab your protein drink later or to skip your lunch to do something for someone else, you jeopardize your own health. Let people know their needs will be met only if you don't have to sacrifice your own health in order to help them.

Action for the day:

Take care of yourself in a healthy way, and then you can help others.

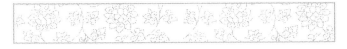

Find your safety zone.

Maybe you're tired and there is too much to do. Perhaps you are the main caretaker of your family. You struggle to keep up with the mess, the appointments, the activities, the laundry, the meals, the schedules, the homework, your job, your sanity, your parents' needs, the bills, the checkbook, the charities, and your spouse. Sometimes you want to scream, but the people around you all look to you for support. They need you to be "together."

You need a place where you can safely go and not be judged—a place where people understand your conflicting desire to help others and to take care of yourself. A place where the other people who supposedly "have it all together" can commiserate with you, laugh with you, or just be with you without judgment. This haven can be a healing place for you. A place of renewal. Sometimes all you need to help you cope is understanding.

Action for the day:

If you don't already have one, meditate on how you might create a safe haven where you can connect with others who will understand and support you.

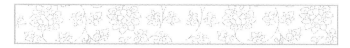

Take small steps.

Visualize the dream come true. You are standing in front of the mirror at your goal weight filled with a sense of accomplishment and purpose. But all big dreams begin with little steps.

To stay on track to reach your dream, try using a daily checklist to monitor your new lifestyle. The checklist is a great tool to keep track of your vitamins, supplements, food choices, exercise, water intake, and mood. Over time, you'll see small victories on your scale and in your life. Maybe you'll fit into an airplane seat or be able to help your kids build a snowman. Let those little victories encourage you to keep using your checklist. Each day that you stay on track brings you closer to the realization of your dream.

Action for the day:

Are you using a checklist? If not, today is a good day to start.

Contribute.

Being obese made your life smaller. You were less able to do even simple activities. You may have spent more time worrying about your woes, rather than figuring out what you could contribute to your community. Following WLS, your energy increases as well as your ability to focus on positive efforts.

Now, you're able to contribute time, energy, and attention outside yourself. Maybe you want to be a foster parent. Or you want to volunteer to help with a cause you've always wished you had the energy and stamina to support. You might just want to bring a meal to a sick friend or help your spouse with the yard work. Whatever you do, approach it with gratitude for your new ability to help others.

Action for the day:

Do something to benefit someone else today.

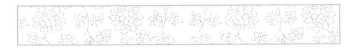

Plan for strong feelings.

After WLS, a flood of feelings may wash over you. Strong emotions can be unsettling. Remember, you are not dealing with feelings the same way anymore. Prior to surgery, you were probably an emotional eater; food was your comfort. Finding ways to control your food intake now may create stress and depression.

You can channel strong emotions in a constructive way. A constructive way is not exchanging one self-destructive behavior for another, like drinking alcohol instead of overeating. Strong emotions do not have to rule you. Recognize them as symptoms of change, and find a way to dispel them without harming yourself or others. And remember, all strong feelings will pass.

Action for the day:

Construct a plan for times when strong feelings arise so that they do not harm you or derail your WLS efforts.

Identify your feelings.

To cope with uncomfortable feelings, you might sometimes choose to overeat, or to eat a food that isn't healthy for you. In the long run, emotional eating can undermine your WLS success.

Mastering your emotional eating will take time, but it is well worth the effort. To start the process, first learn to identify what you are feeling at any given moment.

Action for the day:

Today, do an Internet search for a list of feelings. Print out the list or copy down ten of them that seem most familiar to you. Then, as you go through your day, ask yourself periodically, "What am I feeling at this moment?" Use your new list to help you decide, and be sure to keep a log of your emotions.

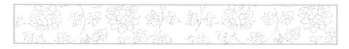

Accept your body.

Are there parts of your body you find so undesirable you hide them from your spouse or significant other? Body image issues are common among weight loss surgery patients. It seems that some people expect perfection in themselves and find any slight flaw a reason for self loathing.

Resources exist to help you loosen the grip a poor body image can have on your life. While you may not love every aspect of your body, you can work on acceptance, and perhaps even learn how to avoid obsessing about your body and how it looks.

Action for the day:

If body image is an issue for you, check out a book from the library about this topic today; or better yet, find a therapist who can help you work through your body image issues.

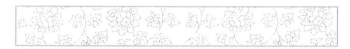

Remind yourself healthy change is worth the discomfort.

To truly get beyond old, unhealthy eating patterns, you will need to change. Accepting that you need to change is the first step. Understanding that change will require you to be uncomfortable for awhile is the next step.

You can help yourself by using positive self talk. Remind yourself frequently that the discomfort you are feeling is temporary, and that eventually your new, healthier behaviors will feel completely normal and comfortable.

Action for the day:

Gently allow yourself to feel the discomfort of change today. Find ways to comfort yourself other than with food. Praise yourself for the effort.

Take charge of your life.

Feeling stuck in life is not uncommon. Maybe you are dealing with circumstances over which you have little control. You feel like you'll never escape.

When you are feeling trapped, it's important to understand the real meaning of the word stuck. For example, it may be less risky to hate your current job than it is to look for a new one. But are you really stuck? Consider the choices you're making. What's holding you back from taking charge? And what are the consequences of not taking charge?

Action for the day:

In your journal, list some areas in your life in which you feel stuck. Pick one area and write honestly about the differences in the cost of staying stuck versus the cost of moving forward.

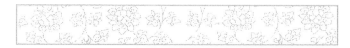

Give your suffering a purpose.

We all have pain and suffering in our lives. What distinguishes us as individuals is how we respond to our suffering. Some people use food, alcohol, shopping, or other addictions to mask the pain. Others live in anger and depression. Some feel an overwhelming sense of self pity.

All of these emotions and coping behaviors are common, but masking the pain does not allow you to overcome it. You have to create purpose for it, or you cannot come to terms with it. When faced with sorrow, you can choose to grow from the experience both emotionally and spiritually. Just know you are not alone in your suffering. What can you do to give your suffering a purpose?

Action for the day:

Meditate on your suffering. How can you use the experience to become a better person? To help others?

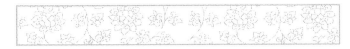

Cook from scratch.

Many people have almost forgotten how to cook a meal from scratch, but cooking from scratch provides myriad benefits.

First, you are moving about the kitchen, so you are undoubtedly burning calories. Second, you can control the quality of the food you use in your cooking, thus boosting the nutritional value. And third, if you're in the kitchen cooking from scratch, you are avoiding the prepared and prepackaged foods that have loads of extra fat (the unhealthy kind) and added sugar (it would surprise you what sugar gets added to!).

Action for the day:

Make a favorite recipe from scratch, substituting lower-fat and whole-grain products for their higher-calorie, refined versions.

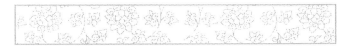

Find your way back.

Just because temptation sometimes wins does not mean all is lost. Giving into temptation does not mean that you have failed or that you are a failure. Everyone strays from the healthy path every now and then. Everyone.

Remember, no matter how far you wander, or how long you wander, you are not forever lost. It may take time to find your way again, but if you strive for willingness, you will find your path. Do not let a little wandering negate the great success you've already had. Even in the middle of a day of grazing, you can change course and get back on track.

Action for the day:

If you have lost your way, ask for directions from someone you trust. Then, follow those directions no matter what.

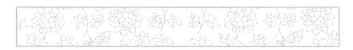

Make your home your sanctuary.

Now that you are living a WLS lifestyle, you have begun to make adjustments in your life. You focus on getting enough protein. You try to eat right and not graze. It's a challenge at times, but you are committed. Sometimes, however, unhealthy foods and old behaviors creep back into your life.

So, make your home your sanctuary. At least there, don't have snack foods sitting out where they call your name every time you walk by. No matter what challenges threaten your WLS success, make your home a fortress against the temptations. Your home is the one place you can have control. Your family may be resistant at first, or they may be angry, but they will adjust. And you are so worth it.

Action for the day:

Walk around your house and make a manageable list of things you will change to make it the sanctuary you need. Today, do one thing on the list.

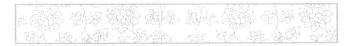

Get connected to your life.

Recovery and healing have as much to do with the mind and
spirit as with the body. Your physical obstacle to relationship
building is being removed day by day. You have the gift of a
new life—a fresh start.

Some people continue to find ways to hide from the world.
If not with weight, then with distraction, obsession, self-
destruction, avoidance, and victimization. You can choose to
learn how to get connected to people and throw off those old
defenses. Study how to love. Study how to give, how to be
safe, how to set boundaries. These studies can be part of your
pursuit to better health. They allow you to heal body, mind,
and spirit.

Action for the day:

Express your love in safe places. If you don't know what or
who is safe, start to learn.

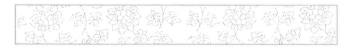

Let go.

The sickness and immobility are gone. You are beginning to
enjoy good health, energy, and hope. It's time to leave your
old habits and old patterns of thinking behind, just as you are
letting go of friends who are no longer good for you. It is
your time to fly.

The ropes that held you down no longer bind you. The only
things holding you to the ground now are your own hands
on the rope. Let go. Be the new person you want to be—the
healthy person who has awakened from a long sickness.

Action for the day:

Meditate on an old behavior, habit, or friend that is no longer
healthy for you. In your journal, write a goodbye letter to
that old behavior or friend. Don't send it. Just experience it.
How does it feel to let go?

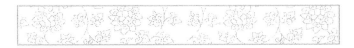

Exercise.

Perhaps you would prefer not to exercise. It takes time, it's
hard, and you don't like to sweat. But even though you can
think of a thousand excuses why you do not want to (or think
you can't) exercise, you know in the long run it will make
you feel better.

At first, exercise can feel like torture, but if you stay vigilant
you will find you become stronger and have more energy.
Exercise also relieves stress. Working out your tensions with
sweat helps to unburden your soul. And you just might find
yourself feeling more cheerful. Prioritize exercise like you
prioritize brushing your teeth, drinking water, or taking your
medicine. For long-term WLS success, it is as essential.

Action for the day: In your journal, make a list of activities
you like to do that involve moving your body. These activities
do not have to be formal exercise. Pick one activity and do
it today.

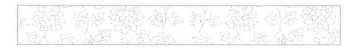

Leave the land of make-believe.

Are you sitting in the land of make-believe, waiting for a handsome prince to rescue you from your problems? Are you wanting to be freed from the castle tower, but don't know how to get out without a fairy godmother or a knight in shining armor?

No matter what your challenge, no matter what is holding you back, you can set yourself free if you put your heart and mind to it. The reality is you can rescue yourself.

Action for the day:

Identify a problem today that has you feeling trapped or hopeless. Then, take some real action toward resolving your problem—even if it's just a small action.

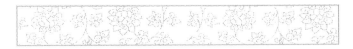

Journal.

Sometimes you may feel you need to sort out your thoughts and feelings, but you really don't want to share them with others. Maybe you feel too vulnerable or too confused. A journal can provide a safe outlet—a private place to think and explore. Putting your thoughts down on paper helps you gain some perspective on your life. A journal will help you remember where you've been, and show you how you've evolved.

Journaling will take you into yourself and help you understand your inner needs and desires. Then, journaling will lead you to a new place by helping you build a foundation from which you can venture out into the world a stronger and more centered person.

Action for the day:

If you haven't done it yet, begin journaling today. If you keep it up, it will change your life—guaranteed.

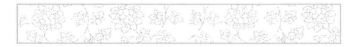

Be spontaneous.

Life has its own energy—a force that drives you through time. You cannot control it; you can only hold on tight and hope not to fall off. You can allow yourself to be frightened by the ride, or you can scream in delight and let yourself be tossed.

Try to roll with the punches, and let things happen as they may. Being flexible and spontaneous is a survival mechanism worth developing. Enjoy the ride of life; fighting the motion will only make you sick.

Action for the day:

When the unpredictable happens, be spontaneous and look for the fun in it.

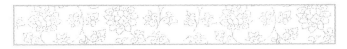

Learn the difference between snacking and grazing.

Snacking and grazing are not the same thing. Snacking has a healthy purpose. You snack because you need a short supply of energy for your body. A snack is planned, including the quality of the food you eat, the quantity, and the time of day. Grazing has no purpose other than to manage emotions or soothe your boredom.

An honest self-assessment should help you determine whether you are snacking or grazing, but if you're not sure ask your nutritionist. Most WLS patients struggle with the urge to graze from time to time, or even most of the time. You can learn strategies to curb grazing, including determining what, if any, planned snack you may need to include in your eating plan. If you are struggling, don't keep it a secret. Ask someone you trust to help you develop the strategies that will work for you.

Action for the day:

Start a food diary today and keep it for three days. Write down what you ate, the time and quantity, and what you were feeling when you ate. Bring this with you the next time you see your nutritionist, and start to explore solutions to your grazing problem.

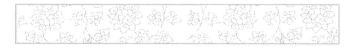

Have courage.

Over time, most people realize they will have to make important changes, difficult changes, if they want long-term WLS success. Some of the changes are physical: more exercise, better eating habits, getting your lab work done regularly. Some of the changes are mental: resolving long-standing depression, changing negative thought patterns, uncovering old ideas that sabotage you. And some of the changes are spiritual: reconnecting with your Creator, learning to care for your soul, and leaving an isolated lifestyle behind.

All these changes are often scary and require hard work. Be brave—physical, mental, and spiritual health await you.

Action for the day:

Take 15 minutes today and make a badge of courage for yourself. Get out the crayons, markers, tape, scissors, glitter...whatever you need. On your badge write something like: "Susan the Brave." Hang your badge where you'll see it every day (and wear it around the house from time to time to help you change how you view yourself and your potential).

Be willing to go to any lengths.

It's not uncommon for a WLS patient to say, "I know I should do that, but I just can't." Drinking water is one such example. Success involves being willing to go to any lengths to achieve your goals. Going to any lengths means doing something you need to do, whether you want to or not, until you have a change of heart and want to do it.

If you can't handle plain water, put mint leaves or cucumber in a jug to flavor it. If you're too busy to drink water, prepare four 16 oz. servings and drink one on the way to work, one during the morning, one during the afternoon, and one on the way home. Use things you do regularly (like driving to and from work) as triggers to drink your water. To say you "can't" is often saying you "won't." Is that how you want to approach this new life you've been given?

Action for the day:

Pick one area in your WLS lifestyle in which you can improve. Today, make the change you need to make, and resolve to keep doing it until you want to do it.

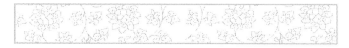

Do the next right thing.

Maybe you haven't scheduled your next follow-up appointment with your WLS surgeon. Or, if you have a band, perhaps you have put off getting the next fill. Maybe you're so busy you have not taken time to connect with your partner or your child.

If you take some time to sit quietly and meditate on what your soul values, you will know what you need to do now. Your life is moving forward fast. Stay focused on moving forward by doing the next right thing today. Support the person you are becoming by attending to your soul.

Action for the day:

Designate a place in your home that is your thinking spot. It must be someplace where you can shut out the world for a little while. Spend five minutes there today checking in with your soul. What is the next right thing you will do?

Be persistent.

Just possessing a skill will not get the job done; you must use your skill over and over again to reach your goal.

Think of the tortoise and hare in Aesop's Fables. The hare was skillful, but not persistent. He stopped and took a nap during the race! But, the tortoise was persistent. He just kept running and running. Slowly and imperfectly, but persistently. Like that brave tortoise, persistent people are rewarded with success. More talented people have fallen short because they did not have the fortitude to go the distance.

Action for the day:

Are you persistent? In your journal, explore how it feels, or would feel, to be persistent and what that might mean for your WLS success.

Distract yourself.

Instead of counting the minutes until the next meal, put something other than food in your mind. Call a friend (you don't have to say why if you don't want to).

Better yet, do something that will make you proud of yourself. Exercise, for instance. Many people hate it, yeah, but when you start substituting something that will make you feel good about yourself (exercise) for something that will depress you (head hunger), you'll, well, feel good about yourself!

Action for the day:

Instead of thinking about food today, find something else to think about. Every time you notice you are obsessing about food, change your focus. Do something to distract yourself.

April

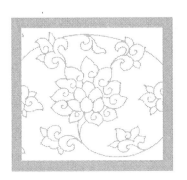

Use all five senses.

Many people who have WLS focus primarily on the sense of
taste for pleasure and soothing. Maybe you know, in theory,
other things would feel good, but food is such an easy and
familiar source of comfort. Finding a new source of pleasure,
and getting as much pleasure from it as you do from eating,
will take time, effort, and open mindedness.

When you accept that food cannot be your only source of
comfort, you make room for other pleasurable experiences.
You can enjoy a delicious massage, listen to motivating music,
appreciate a beautiful painting, or relax with aromatherapies.

Action for the day:

Today, think about other pleasures in life besides food. Try
something enjoyable that involves a sense other than taste.
Don't be afraid to take a risk.

Strike back.

Decadent desserts grace the covers of magazines in the checkout lane, not to mention the array of candy displayed there. Everything is super-sized, and tantalizing smells fill the air. We are encouraged to eat seconds, and how can we pass on dessert? And what about the well-meaning person who declares, "One bite won't hurt."?

Yes, it will! The world will try to sabotage your efforts. From the spouse that leaves food lying around the house to the person pushing samples at the grocery store, you are under attack. Your armor is your resolve, and your mouth is your sword. When the saboteur strikes, strike back with these powerful words: "No, thank you."

Action for the day:

Develop a strategy to deal with the abundance of food surrounding you—write it down in your journal. Make some guidelines by which you can sustain your new life. Review them often.

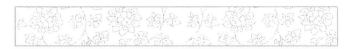

Journey toward total health.

When the soul is troubled, the body suffers one way or another. You will be whole when you find serenity within. Work toward an inner peace, a quiet strength. Strive to accept those things you cannot change.

As you journey, choose to love your life and yourself at a deeper level. Take comfort in the fact that your WLS has set your endeavor in motion. You are getting healthier physically and mentally. By finding joy in each success, you nurture your soul as well as your body.

Action for the day:

Today, choose to love your life. Reflect on how you can find peace through loving acceptance. For example, you can love your career for the people you work with, what you do, what you produce, or just because it provides the resources to do what you want to do.

Channel stress.

Remember studying the "fight or flight" mechanism? Stress produces adrenaline in animals, as when they face their predators in the wild, so they will have the strength to fight or to run if necessary.

Stress produces adrenaline in humans also, only we can't fight or run. Instead, we experience unyielding stress! Your dilemma is: Do you channel this stress energy into frustration and anger or do you use it to power a solution? People who perform magnificently under stress have mastered the art of channeling the energy positively. They have adopted an attitude about stress that is beneficial to them, rather than letting stress...well...stress them out! Stress is an energy you can use to accomplish what needs to be done.

Action for the day:

Use stress to your advantage today. Work through it to accomplish a task. Adopt the attitude that stress is energy to be channeled.

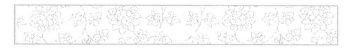

Take control.

Are you in control of your life or does addiction, in one form or another, control you? When you are in control, you can decide to stop an unwanted behavior, and there is little consequence. It's a simple decision.

If you have trouble stopping your behavior, and you can't seem to get it out of your mind, you may be facing an addiction. You may find yourself obsessing, or even suffering withdrawal symptoms (such as nervousness, sweating, or excessive anxiety). When you experience withdrawal, you have crossed a line. You are not in control anymore. If you get to that point, you must seek out help.

Action for the day:

Evaluate if you are obsessing about something. Decide who will be in control—you or your obsession. If you need help, get it.

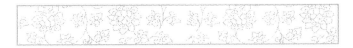

Fake it till you make it.

Your life has changed dramatically in a short period of time. Whereas your days prior to surgery probably consisted more of survival techniques than anything else, your life post surgery embraces new opportunities.

Do you treat your new life as an opportunity or as a challenge? Do you face each moment with hope? Do you encourage yourself with words like, "I am getting better every day in every way?" Do you face each moment with confidence knowing that each challenge you overcome makes you stronger and healthier? Resolve to believe in your abilities today.

Action for the day:

Today is a "fake-it-till-you-make-it" day. Act as if you are confident and hopeful. Sometimes this new attitude takes quite a bit of practice, but eventually you WILL make it.

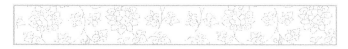

Live the life you've got.

How many people go through life wishing for something they don't have? Do you live for the future? Some people have feelings of longing for years, then come to regret what they missed because they were always wishing away their life.

You define your life through your choices. Sometimes the choice is to live well the life you've been dealt. Count your blessings and appreciate the richness of your life. Avoid counting the things you don't have. Live your life, with all its imperfections. It is yours. Work at it. Appreciate it. Craft it into a life you really want by living each moment to the fullest—no matter where you are on your life journey.

Action for the day:

Today, work on accepting your life as it is. Only then can you begin to live it fully here and now.

Respect yourself.

If your self image is built on self respect, and not on the
tenuous respect of others, then you are invincible. When you
base how you feel about yourself on what others think, then
you go into the world vulnerable. And no one gets through
this life without criticism or unkind words directed at them
from time to time. No one.

Be yourself. Be the person you want to be. Be a person you
can respect. How do you do that? Identify your values and
live by them. When you develop a track record of meeting
your own standards, then no matter what negative comments
come your way, they bounce off you and you are not so
deeply hurt. People treat each other poorly out of jealousy
and out of their own poor self image. When someone puts
you down, they are attempting to elevate themselves.
Don't let them get to you.

Action for the day:

In your journal, make a list of your values and the standards
by which you want to live. Work on living up to your own
ideals. Impress only yourself.

Honor yourself.

Dignity comes from the image we have of ourselves,
knowing what we are worth. It does not come from society's
recognition of us. The most honored person in society will
possess no dignity unless she considers herself worthy.

We honor ourselves with what we do and how we respect
ourselves. We have a right to be proud of our accomplishments and thankful for coming this far. This self honor
is dignity.

Action for the day:

Honor yourself today. In your journal, make a list of your
recent accomplishments. If your list is short, do something
today you can add to that list.

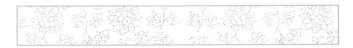

Embrace normalcy.

In your life after WLS, you have focused on yourself. You have undergone changes in your body, diet, and environment. Maybe you've been noticed and praised a bit. People are talking to you, holding doors, looking you in the eye. Maybe you're feeling more confident. Sometimes you feel like the center of attention. Soon the attention may lessen. You reach goal and become just an ordinary person again. New people you meet don't even know you were ever obese.

Life will resume as it did before. The end of the joy ride can be a big let down. The great test is to try not to become that center again. Enjoy being a regular person with common experiences to share with others. The roller coaster ride is over, and the real journey to wellness has begun.

Action for the day:

Work on accepting that your time as the center of attention passes; it is a part of life not a statement of who you are. Today, make an effort to be a friend among friends, not the star.

Face your truth.

If you are finding that you don't want to do the things that will keep you healthy, it's time to pull out your tool kit. For example, go back to your support group. Call another WLS patient who may need support. Ask a friend to exercise with you. But most importantly, be honest with yourself. Sometimes WLS patients start to slip into old behaviors and the consequences are not immediately apparent. Sadly, the consequences appear down the road when damage has already been done.

Denial can cause serious damage. The truth will protect you— if you will embrace it. What is the truth about where you are in your WLS journey today? Are you doing everything you need to do?

Action for the day:

In your journal create a contract with yourself (and don't forget to sign it!). State the action you are committing to. Be specific. Include dates, times, amounts, whatever information you need to track your progress.

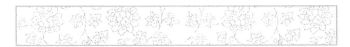

Stop.

Much of the tension in life is due to the fact that people rarely stop doing things. We never give ourselves a break to relieve the tensions of the day, to just do nothing and see where it leads us. Do you feel like you never have a moment when you are not running or in demand? Take time to relax.

And remember, sleeping at night does NOT count as relaxing. Relaxing is being awake and unstressed. It is occupying yourself happily with something you love to do or nothing at all!

Action for the day:

Set aside time to relax and "do nothing" today, even if for a short while. Even five minutes of down time can be replenishing.

Practice curiosity.

Boredom is one of the main reasons people overeat. You have nothing to do, so you migrate to the kitchen and rummage for food. Or your hands are idle while you are reading or watching TV, and you decide to snack.

Curiosity is a great tool to deal with boredom. Have you noticed that when your mind is busy looking into something, it banishes thoughts of eating? If you are searching for an answer, the obsession keeps your mind busy. Find a subject or hobby that excites you and make it your new obsession. Whatever you choose, it will liberate you. Overcome the need to eat when bored by becoming curious.

Action for the day:

Choose a topic or activity about which you are curious and research it today. Except at mealtime, focus on your new interest instead of food. Practice curiosity.

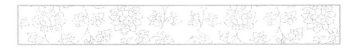

Share, don't compare.

Do you think other people have more fun than you? More stuff? An easier life? That is not always true. Most everyone has problems and challenges, just like you. It may seem that everyone else is doing better with their weight loss. You may think they look better or are having an easier time of things.

Maybe they are struggling with something like temptation, forgetfulness, or missing their vitamins or protein. It's commonplace for people to put on a good face in public—they create an illusion. Try not to compare yourself to others. Comparisons serve no healthy purpose. You are on your own journey. This is the time to band together with others who are on a similar path and share support. Share, don't compare.

Action for the day:

Resolve to accept where you are on your journey, and don't compare yourself to others today. Instead, get support and plan your next steps—striving for progress, not perfection.

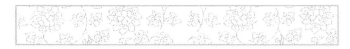

Redefine yourself.

One of the keys to long-term success is to change the way you view yourself. If you are a "fat person" who has lost weight, your subconscious is likely to work on regaining your "fat person" status.

If you are a "health-conscious, energetic person" your subconscious will strive for that state. It's not just semantics. It's the truth. Redefining yourself and believing your new definition takes time and effort. But this process is critical to your success.

Action for the day:

In your journal, write for five minutes on who you are. Try to uncover some of the negative views you have, such as "I am worthless," or "I'm too set in my ways to change," or "I'm too busy to live the WLS lifestyle." Once you've identified your old definition, spend five minutes writing a new one. Start living according to your new definition.

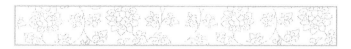

Have fun now; it's later than you think.

Fun is not only for children. Fun can be found by anyone in any moment of the day. Having fun is a choice. Even at the most horrible job, fun can be had if it is just imagining bunny ears growing out of the boss's head.

Laughter will lift your spirits and keep you young. It will improve your health. Find fun where you can. Write a note to stick in your child's or spouse's lunch bag. Have spice tea instead of plain. Spontaneously tickle someone you love. Buy flowers. Do things you know will make you smile.

Action for the day:

What are you waiting for? If your life is nothing to smile about, spend some time reviewing your typical day. How can you add some fun? Make a list of things (small and large) that you can do to inject fun into your life.

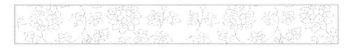

Switch your focus from desire to gratitude.

So many times we whine about what we don't have. Yet, if we had all that we wished for we would probably have more than we could handle. Most of us have more than we need, and many of us have more than we will need in a lifetime. Are you thankful for what you have?

Each day is a gift. Each day you wake up under a roof with clothes to wear, enough food to eat, and electricity, makes you richer than most people in the world. But, despite what you have, do you desire more? Of course we are deserving of all that we have, and desires are motivating. Your desires inspire you to take on challenges and enrich your being. But when your desires leave you blind to the things you already have, and you begin to live for what you don't have—you aren't living well. Be thankful for what you have, and thankful for your desires that can motivate you in a healthy way.

Action for the day:

Today in your journal, make a new gratitude list. You just can't write too many of these mood-changing lists!

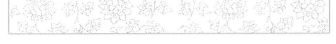

Hear what is not said.

Our loved ones want to be supportive, but may hesitate at times to speak their minds. Observe body language and behavior cues to learn what others are thinking. They may have unspoken questions, concerns, or comments. Even coworkers may not want to upset your "fragile" frame of mind by saying or doing anything "wrong."

Your surgery and inconsistent eating habits may cause others to feel as though they are walking on egg shells. You may think everyone has adjusted to your new lifestyle, but they may just be acting that way to please you. Continue to open lines of communication with your spouse, children, and coworkers so that they are clear about boundaries—both theirs and yours.

Action for the day:

Spend some time today thinking about how your WLS journey affects those around you. Do you need to communicate better with your family, friends, and coworkers? What needs to be said that you haven't said? What do others need you to understand, even if they can't find the words to tell you?

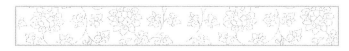

Set new goals.

Has your WLS routine become almost second nature, like brushing your teeth? Do you have some spare time and energy now that you've gotten used to your new life? What are you doing with this new-found energy? Do you feel restless?

If so, this restlessness is a beacon of achievement. You are no longer content to sit and direct life from a chair. You want to jump in and figure out what to conquer next. This is the signal to set some goals. By setting goals you will start to see a path, complete with obstacles that must be overcome. Setting several goals, in different areas of your life, helps you avoid having nothing to do after you've completed one. Revel in your new-found energy, and channel it to achieve goals that were once only dreams. Expand your life as you shrink your body. And take some risks.

Action for the day:

Restlessness is not a signal for despair, but rather action. In your journal, write down a short list of goals encompassing several areas of your life: body, mind, spirit, relationships, health, finances, career, etc.

View permanent weight loss as a process, not an event.

Most great achievements are the result of hard work and a designated plan of action. As they are often time consuming, progress is made in small, purposeful steps.

The same is true concerning permanent weight loss. It's not just going to happen. Through a process you create and execute, you are infinitely more likely to succeed in all your endeavors. Save the "events" for birthdays and celebrations, and view permanent weight loss as a process of making a plan, and then, each day, doing the next right thing.

Action for the day:

Today, simply do the next right thing. Whenever you have a decision to make, whether it's what to eat or what to do after work, do the next right thing.

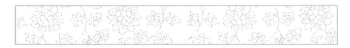

Rethink your goal weight.

A common attitude for many WLS patients is, "My surgeon said I should weigh about 150 pounds, but I want to weigh 135—the weight I was when I graduated from high school."

While common, the desire to get down to a number you have assigned meaning to, whether the number is realistic or not, may sabotage your long-term weight loss. Your ideal weight is more a matter of the intersection between the sustainable lifestyle choices you make and how your body responds to weight loss surgery. Consider giving yourself permission to let your body weigh what it wants to weigh, with you eating and exercising at the healthiest levels you can sustain.

Action for the day:

Rethink your goal weight. Is it realistic? Is it sustainable? If you are not sure, do some research. Talk to your doctor and nutritionist. Then make a decision based on the knowledge you gain.

Take care of your "tool."

A carpenter uses a router to carve beautiful designs and to make notches to piece furniture together. Yet if he does not know how to use this tool, he only destroys the wood he is carving.

The same holds true with your stomach pouch. If you care for it by following your surgeon's guidelines, your tool will perform well for you. However, gastric bypass patients who continually eat more than their pouch can comfortably hold may stretch the stoma or opening from the stomach to the intestines. Lapband patients may avoid getting a needed fill or may eat too many soft, rich foods, thus making their tool ineffective.

Action for the day:

Review your surgeon's instructions. Are you using your pouch well?

Avoid the foods that do you in.

What, if any, foods trigger negative emotions in you? Do
you crave certain foods? Are there foods that make you
feel deprived? These foods are the ones to avoid as much
as possible.

No one is perfect, but the people who succeed at lasting
weight loss are the ones who understand how certain foods
negatively affect them and eliminate those foods from their
diet. Try to be honest with yourself as you examine your
feelings during meals.

Action for the day:

In your journal, write down how you feel about this day's
inspiration. Do any foods come to mind that you need to
consider eliminating from your diet?

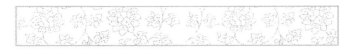

Be sensitive to how your changes affect others.

People may not understand why you have made so many changes that affect their lives. A spouse may be confused by your new interests. Your friend may miss having her eating buddy on Friday nights. Your boss may not understand your moodiness as you adjust to your new lifestyle. Your kids may miss getting fast food.

Let others know you understand your changes affect them. Tell your children, for example, you will be able to play with them more because you will be healthier. Explain to your husband that you want to be more active with him, rather than watch TV. Try to help people adjust to your new way of being.

Action for the day:

Discuss the affects of your changes with others who are close to you.

Avoid martyrdom.

How many times have you sat down with friends at a dinner party for a lovely meal and someone who has never had a weight problem goes on and on about how they can't eat this or that because they are on a diet? As a result, at least some people at the table felt self conscious about filling their plate and enjoying their meal. Not only did the "dieter" spoil the meal, but they openly insulted the host by judging the dinner unfit to eat.

The middle of a dinner party is not the best time to share your personal choices and to become a martyr for your new lifestyle. You can take your smaller portions and not draw attention to them. If someone asks you why you took so little, just say you want to sample everything, and then change the subject. Be a rounded conversationalist, and people will remember the interesting person they sat next to as opposed to the person who made them feel bad about themselves.

Action for the day:

Reflect on ways to be interesting around people instead of focusing everyone's attention on your food choices.

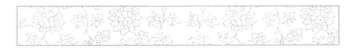

Listen to your intuition.

How many times have you jumped into a decision without thinking it through? Have you ever made a decision because you wanted to get it over with, even though deep down you knew something was not quite right?

It's hard to quiet down and listen to the inner voice that tells you when you are rushing a decision or ignoring a nagging thought about it. Not all bad outcomes can be avoided, but the ones that could have been—if only you had listened to your inner voice—are particularly painful.

Action for the day:

Be clear about your decisions. If you have hesitation or doubt, listen to those feelings today. Most decisions really don't have to be rushed.

Struggle and win.

One day it may be so easy to do everything right you don't even need to think, whereas the next day everything is an effort. When you face a difficult day, it's easy to want to give up, yet this might be the day that breaks the plateau or the day you reach the next milestone. To give up at this point, when you have come so far, is not an option.

Even though your goal may be far away, struggling one more step gets you closer. When the labor of the day is too much, turn to your support—a person, a book, a quote, or your higher power (or all of these things). Cling to the support you have to help you take the next step toward your goal. Much later, after you have met your goal, you'll appreciate the struggle for having made you stronger.

Action for the day:

Days of struggle are bound to happen, but help is not far away. Today, reach for that help whenever you need it.

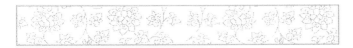

Be a little self-centered.

With WLS, to become a little self-centered is a healthy
survival mechanism. You need to meet your needs on a very
specific basis and must schedule the rest of life around
those needs as best you can.

It's easy to allow other things to take precedence over your
WLS needs. But, please be firm with yourself on this. It's very
common to want to put others first, but you risk permanent
health complications when you do things like put off taking
vitamins or delay getting your lab work done.

Action for the day:

If your post-WLS health regimen is lacking, make it your
mission to find out why. Is it because you're putting everyone
else's needs before your own?

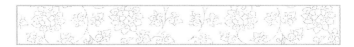

Prioritize, prioritize, prioritize.

We need to eat. We need to bathe. We need to sleep. We need to pay bills and run errands. And then, WLS brings even more needs into our lives—like taking vitamins and protein supplements, exercising, and getting lab work done. These things are not really choices for WLS patients, they are priorities. Do you put off the things you need to be doing?

The greatest excuse of the procrastinator is, "I forgot." When you write down your needs and refer to the list often, you can't forget. Maybe what you really mean is, "I don't want to." The best response to that is, "You have to. This is not a choice. I can make you do it." Allow your inner parent to say this to the child inside you who is rebelling.

Action for the day:

Are you rebelling? In your journal, make a list of the things you need to do—the things that, in all honesty, are not optional. Use your new list as a checklist to motivate you.

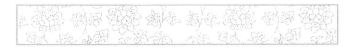

Examine your friendships.

Friendships endure when mutual respect and support for each other is the foundation. A healthy friendship tends to stick even as people change. Other friendships cannot survive when people make major life changes. If the relationship was based on shared, self-destructive behavior, like overeating, when the behavior isn't shared anymore, the relationship loses its foundation and crumbles.

It may be time to let go of an unhealthy friendship. In some instances, it will be painful to lose the relationship. You may feel lonely for a time. In other instances you may just move on, remembering your old friend fondly. You will find new friends; such is the path of life. Have no regrets for moving on to new, healthier relationships.

Action for the day:

Today, evaluate your friendships. Are you holding on to people who aren't right for you anymore? Have courage, and if you need to—let go.

May

Stay current.

You may be sick of reading up on the topics of WLS, nutrition, and exercise. But, continuing your education in these areas is important. Research on those topics is ongoing. New discoveries are being made daily; for example, unexpected vitamin deficiencies recently were discovered in some WLS patients.

Each phase of your recovery has its own problems and pitfalls. It's easy to get into the mindset that you know it all and become less vigilant about your health. Staying current on WLS-related topics only reinforces the good habits you have already mastered and introduces you to possible new ways to maintain your success.

Action for the day:

Look up something new about WLS or research a question you have yet to answer.

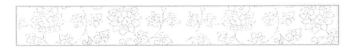

Automate your life.

WLS and the self care it demands are but one facet of your life. Your self care can be looked at like breathing—something that is necessary to your life, but that you do without thinking, automatically. You don't stop breathing while you work, yet you don't take time to think about breathing either: Expand diaphragm, take in air, relax diaphragm, let air out, repeat.

The same principle can apply to your WLS lifestyle. Make it as automatic as possible. If you are fearful of forgetting the time and missing your meal or protein, use a timer or alarm of some kind. That leaves your brain free to do other things. Keep your water bottle in view and you will reach for it more often. Small adjustments can help incorporate your self care into your life. WLS is a part of your life, not your whole life.

Action for the day:

Are there strategies you can apply to make living with WLS more automatic? Take some time today to make your WLS lifestyle easier to manage.

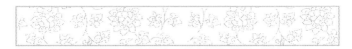

Understand worry is a waste of time.

Have you ever avoided doing something because you
were worried about what might happen if you did it? Living
according to your worries can create problems, because
worries deal with what might happen, not what will happen.

If your worries paralyze you, remember that nothing bad or
good will happen without action. You'll never know what
might be unless you take some risk. It's true, consequences
will occur as a result of your actions, but that's not always a
bad thing. Worries only serve to hold you back from reaching
your potential. Casting them aside, you'll find the reality is
usually much more tolerable than the imagined.

Action for the day:

Are worries holding you back and controlling your life?
In your journal, make a list of your main worries and explore
how you can move past them.

Accept that you are human and are going to fall at times.

How you act after you fall determines your fate. Sooner or later you will eat something you feel is "wrong." Maybe you'll eat something unplanned at a party, or drive through to get an old favorite when you're in a hurry. After a stumble, pick yourself up, dust yourself off, and start over—without looking back and without guilt.

You can waste a lot of energy feeling angry and guilty for not being perfect. Understand that these cravings and feelings are normal and have nothing to do with personal strength or resolve. You cannot allow these feelings to crush your spirit. In fact, a poor food choice is simply a signal you need to make a positive choice as soon as possible. Starting over (and over and over, if necessary) is looking forward to success, instead of dwelling on mistakes.

Action for the day:

Start over today and move on. Instead of kicking yourself for a poor choice, focus on how great your next choice will be.

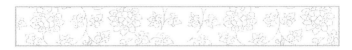

Create a new and improved community.

A support network is vital to your success. So, embrace or create a community of supporters who will nurture you throughout your life. Surround yourself with people who love you for who you are, and who will be there for you no matter what. Do business with competent professionals who treat you with respect and good will. Nurture friendships with people who do not base their friendship with you on who they need you to be for them.

Your family can't be chosen, so limit your exposure with family members who are not supportive of your new lifestyle. Spend as much time as possible with people who encourage you. When you add a new person to your community, consider them carefully. This healthy community you are building is for your life.

Action for the day:

Review your relationships. Have you built a supportive and loving community? If not, in your journal, make a list of things you can do to begin that process. Do one thing on your list today.

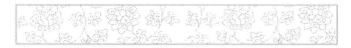

Give a gift to yourself.

How often do you go through your day doing what you have
to do, rather than doing what excites you? Sometimes people
who have been chronically ill with obesity have spent years
trying to comfort themselves with food and have not explored
other areas of pleasure. Maybe chronic pain or depression
held them back.

But now you can learn, maybe for the first time, what feels
good to you. Really good. Luxurious. Deeply satisfying.
Comforting. Nurturing. Soothing. Self loving. Totally
relaxing. Exciting. What satisfies you deeply? It might be
incorporating a new color into your décor. It might be music.
It might be planting a sweet-smelling flower. Give yourself
the gift of pleasure in life that extends beyond what you eat.

Action for the day:

Spend the day paying attention to what feels good. Reflect
on this simple yet important truth. Do something that really
excites you today.

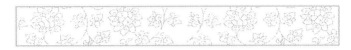

Make restaurants safe and enjoyable.

Eating a meal in a restaurant does not have to bring you guilt and remorse. It can be a great experience with the right attitude and tools. Some people order a "to go" box when they place their order. When the meal arrives they put about 1/2 in the box and save it for another meal.

You can delay eating. Don't begin eating the minute the appetizer is put on the table. Wait awhile and enjoy the conversation. You also can cut your food into very small pieces. Eat each bite slowly, and chew, chew, chew. That alone will leave you feeling full and satisfied, while having had appropriate portions.

Action for the day:

Practice the tool of cutting small bites, and chewing slowly and thoroughly. You might find your meals even more satisfying when you savor your food this way.

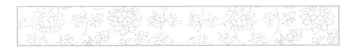

Be patient.

We've all dreamt about "The Day"—the glorious morning when we step on the scale and that magic number blinks into view. And having WLS was a BIG, exciting step toward that goal.

But eventually, the novelty wore off, right? And as you settled into your daily routine, your journey began to seem tedious. Perhaps your weight loss slowed or you hit a plateau. If depression and despair threaten your goals, remember that patience is the key.

Action for the day:

Parenting, like other life journeys, is often described as a "marathon" rather than a "sprint." Today, have a mini-marathon of your own. Take a walk around the neighborhood, but instead of turning it into a workout, force yourself to slow down and enjoy the outdoors. And if there happen to be roses along your path, be sure to take a whiff.

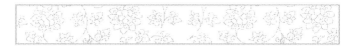

Commit to action.

You've probably heard the phrase "Don't put off until tomorrow what you can do today." Yes, it's a cliché, but it rings exceptionally true for WLS patients.

It's frighteningly easy to put your health on the back burner. Maybe you get so busy during the day that you think nothing of skipping meals or forgetting to drink your water. Of course, one day won't matter in the long run, but by putting things off until "tomorrow" you're really telling yourself that you're not worth the time and effort it would take to care for your health. Because the funny thing about waiting for tomorrow is...we put the tasks off until tomorrow, again.

Action for the day:

If you've been letting other things get in the way of your WLS lifestyle, take action TODAY to get back on track. Sign up for an exercise class, create a supplement regimen, or start keeping a journal of what you eat.

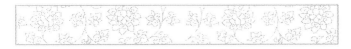

Gas up.

Like any machine, your body functions only as well as you treat it. It needs healthy "fuel" to run smoothly, and if it doesn't get it, it becomes sluggish. Just as a machine rusts and freezes up when it is not used, the body stiffens and atrophies.

Consider your own situation: Has improper maintenance been your policy for years? Do you feed your mood even when the food is counter to what your body needs? When you feed your body the right fuel, your mood improves and your body is healthier for it.

Action for the day:

Keep a food journal for a few days. Notice how your body feels when you feed it well.

Turn a negative into a positive.

Many WLS patients have such a poor self-image they spend their time looking for flaws in those around them: The thin saleswoman has a crooked nose…your rich friend's children are badly behaved…your pretty sister has awful hair.

But consider this: If you do not find the beauty in everything, praise people genuinely for their accomplishments, and wish good will on others, how can you expect to learn to love and accept yourself? When you are a person who always has a kind word, can always see beauty, and is genuinely happy for another's success, then you will see the beauty in yourself. You will know joy.

Action for the day:

Today, notice your thoughts and judgments. Whenever you have a critical thought, replace it with a loving thought.

Allow yourself to experience emotions.

Some of us have been so hurt and tortured by our pasts that we have built walls up to protect ourselves. We have shut down our emotions, knowing if we can't feel something, it can't hurt us. But if you cut yourself off from the possibility of being hurt, you also close yourself to the possibility of feeling positive emotions like love and joy.

Let other people in. Open your heart and spirit to people who genuinely care for you and support your new lifestyle. These people are less likely to let you down or to hurt you. And when you do get hurt (because eventually you will), learn to communicate your feelings to the person whose words or deeds were painful to you. You can create a deeply fulfilling new life by opening yourself up to emotions.

Action for the day:

Do you wall off your emotions to avoid being hurt? In your journal, write a letter to your emotions. Encourage them to come out, gently. As always, seek counsel when you need it.

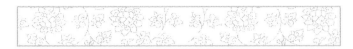

Set the bar low.

Some days you will wake up and spring out of bed ready to exercise and some days you won't. In fact, some weeks or months you'll feel motivated and some you won't. But no matter how you feel, you know you must exercise. So what do you do when you don't want to?

Set the bar low. Tell yourself you only have to stretch today. Or that you only have to exercise for 5 minutes. Don't worry about the intensity and duration on a bad day, just worry about showing up. Motivation follows action, even when it's only a little action.

Action for the day:

If you are feeling resistant to exercise today, set a timer for 5 minutes and march in place or do stretches. Just do something.

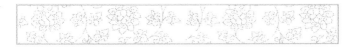

Learn maintenance.

Maintenance is one of the more scary things for people who struggle with weight. Many people fear they will simply give up or become complacent. And of course, there is the fear of gaining all your weight back and more. The idea of maintaining your weight year after year can be daunting. It may even feel boring.

Are you afraid you'll fail at maintenance? Have courage. Maintenance is a skill you can learn. For example, you can weigh yourself once a week and if you are up a pound or two, follow your program religiously until the next time you weigh. If you are still up a bit, talk to your nutritionist and make minor adjustments to your diet, or exercise a bit more. Making little changes when necessary and keeping faith in yourself will help you sort out how to maintain.

Action for the day:

If you have not reached a maintenance weight, spend some time thinking about and planning for maintenance. How will you handle it? If you are at your maintenance weight, evaluate how you are doing and make small adjustments as necessary.

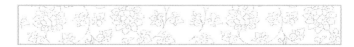

Practice restraint.

We live in a world of abundance. Everywhere we go we have choices. Stores are filled with things we want, whether we need them or not. And, of course, delectable foods are everywhere. American culture teaches you that you deserve to have what you want, when you want it.

Try taking a cue from your grandparents: They were raised in a different era. They had to save up for things, conserve things, go without. Sometimes taking a look at others' hardships can make it easier to face our own.

Action for the day:

Just for today, practice restraint. Deny yourself something you want, and think positive thoughts about your choice. For example, say to yourself, "I'm not going to buy a latte today because I want to learn restraint, and I will love how much better I feel when that happens."

Know your limits.

Are you starting to feel unstoppable? Do you have more
energy than you have had in years? You may feel like you can
almost fly, that you can run forever…but will you be in pain
the next day?

You may believe that the only way to get to the next fitness
level is through experiencing intense pain. But hurting
yourself by pushing past your limits can actually hamper
your workout routine, rather than enhancing your fitness.
Consistent exercise will serve you much better than sporadic,
painful exercise. Your body knows what it can do; listen to it
and stop when you've hit your limit, so that you can remain
consistent.

Action for the day:

Evaluate your exercise routine. Are you pushing too hard?
If you are left feeling depleted, rather than fatigued, after
exercise, you might want to consider slowing down a bit.
Consistency is key.

Love yourself unconditionally.

Regrettably, some people battling obesity feel they are unworthy of love. Years of negative comments have made them feel unlovable—even though that is not the case.

Perhaps you have spent so many years hating your outer self that you can no longer see any inward beauty. Your self-worth is not dependant on your outward appearance. Own this concept today! Do not hesitate to break down those beliefs of worthlessness.

Action for the day:

Think of someone who loves you absolutely, and take a peek at yourself through that person's eyes. If you still can't see, ask that person directly to share the beauty they see in you. Don't worry about appearances; you're not being narcissistic. This is about your emotional healing—about finally recognizing the beauty that is in you.

Break the rules.

Some days it's hard to do the right thing. You don't want to eat your protein or drink your water. Maybe you just don't feel like exercising. That's normal. If it's a rare event to want to "rebel" against your routine, then you're probably okay. Give yourself a small break. But when the days of rebellion start to add up, you're in trouble. How do you cope with rebellious feelings? Sometimes the easiest thing to do is break down your "have-tos" into a checklist. Then, cross off or modify things that are truly non-essential. For example, you may want to exercise, but do you have to go running? Maybe cleaning your house or walking at the mall will check off the exercise box a little less painfully.

The action you take in the face of rebellion isn't as important as having a strategy for dealing with it. Plan for rebellion, rather than letting it take over your life.

Action for the day:

In your journal, write your step-by-step "Rebellion Action Plan." What will you do the next time you don't want to follow your routine?

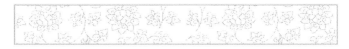

Pass it on.

New people join WLS support groups. You may run into them at WLS-related appointments. You might even meet them by referral. People new to WLS need a mentor just like you did. They are as frightened and unsure as you were. By sharing your transformation, you can be a blessing to them on their own journey.

You can help them find the perfect-tasting protein shake or help them shop for the best foods. Invite them to join your exercise group. Some people have not participated in group exercise, and may be anxious about trying it. Newcomers need mentors, supporters, and friends. WLS patients who reach out to the next "generation" WLS patients tend to do better with their own recovery and progress.

Action for the day:

Today, reach out to a newcomer. For example, go to your hospital and visit a bariatric patient. Share your experiences with them and make them feel welcome in this new world.

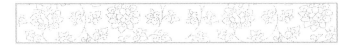

Carpe diem.

It may sound cliché, but seizing the day as a WLS patient keeps you in the present. Try not to revert to old habits and your old flawed thinking. Really take a hold of this day and LIVE it. Appreciate each moment that makes up this day, and do an activity you would not have been able to perform prior to WLS.

What a gift you have been given with WLS! Celebrate today and the opportunity you have been given to reclaim your life.

Action for the day:

Have fun! Remember the physical restrictions that applied to the old you? Pick an activity today that would have been difficult to do in the past. Ride a bike, go for a walk, garden. Whatever it is—seize this moment in time.

Be honest with yourself.

People who have WLS generally lose between 60 and 80 percent of their excess weight. Also, people often regain about 10 to 15 pounds. Being honest with yourself means identifying and accepting a weight that you can live with, even if it doesn't match that "magic number" on the scale.

If you have regained 10 to 15 pounds (or have not lost at least 60 percent of your excess weight within 18 months after surgery), it's time to take an honest look at your program. Most people know what they are doing that is sabotaging their weight-loss success. But it's important to keep in mind that on rare occasion a physical reason may impede your efforts such as a staple-line disruption. So, if you are "doing everything right" and still struggling with weight, talk to your surgeon.

Action for the day:

Keep a food, mood, and exercise log this week. You don't have to do it forever, just this week. You'll be surprised at what you learn.

Don't let the world steal your peace.

So much is happening in today's world. Watching the news
can be very upsetting. If you've already had a challenging day,
the violence of a TV show may add more stress. Sometimes
people don't realize how much their environment and what
they allow into their lives affects them.

If you are having trouble with stress eating, or even if you just
feel a lot of stress, consider the impact of the media in your
life. Do you have to read in your local paper about the recent
murders or car accidents? Do you have to watch the news and
see the graphic violence taking place around the world?
Setting good boundaries includes deciding what you want to
be exposed to on a daily basis.

Action for the day:

Spend today noticing how well you control your environment
and what you allow into your life. Are there boundaries you
can set for yourself to bring more peace into your life?

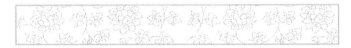

Practice self honesty.

Are you acknowledging to yourself that you are not on track with some or all of your WLS guidelines? For example, are you tracking your weight so that you'll know if you start to gain? Or have you started eating a food item that has been a trigger food in the past?

Self honesty is a critical tool for WLS success. Because WLS requires you to change old thinking and old behaviors, you will benefit from honest self reflection. If you won't admit to yourself what your problems are, how can you possibly solve them?

Action for the day:

For today, spend a few minutes taking a personal inventory. Are you following your WLS guidelines? What problems do you need to solve? Write about this in your journal.

Use a food plan, not a diet.

Even after WLS, it's tempting to remain in a "diet mentality."
It's easy to obsess about the scale and decide how you are
going to feel each day based on that. It's easy to restrict what
you're eating a little more than your food plan calls for. It's
easy to skip meals.

Structured eating can be very helpful to people who have had
WLS. It's helpful to plan what you are going to eat, how
much, and when. That way you can assure yourself you are
getting the nutrition you need. Dieting, on the other hand,
can undermine your success. Dieting can trigger an overeating
"rebound," and it can cause you to restrict too much and halt
your weight loss.

Action for the day:

To the best of your ability, use a food plan today that feeds
you enough, but not too much or too little. If you are unsure
about what quantity to have, talk to your nutritionist.

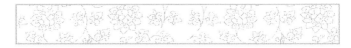

Exercise your mind.

"Exercising" your mind is just as important as strengthening your body. In fact, you can do both at the same time. Some people get bored with their exercise routine, and adding something to keep their mind busy is just the thing to keep them motivated.

The tedium of an exercise routine will bore the mind if it is not inspired on a regular basis. You can exercise your mind through meditation, books on tape, brainstorming, prayer, or socialization (exercising with a friend).

Action for the day:

Today, find a way to exercise your mind while you are exercising your body. Plan what you will do with your mind so that boredom doesn't sabotage your exercise.

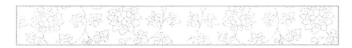

Avoid the pit.

Imagine a deep pit. At the bottom of this pit is a collection of horrors: shards of glass, discarded barb wire, filthy water, poisonous water snakes, and toxic waste. It's deadly down there! The best strategy is to stay far away from the edge.

When you were obese, you might have felt as horrible as if you had been thrown into that pit of despair, only your collection of horrors was pain, hopelessness, and illness. But now, despite the horrors of obesity still fresh in your mind, are you living at the edge of that pit? Is it worth the risk?

Action for the day:

Are you living on the edge? Keeping candy or other refined foods in your house, eating out too much, baking for other people, or drinking with your meals? Think about how you can move away from the edge. Today, take a step away from that horrible pit.

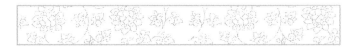

Make your health a priority.

Many people tend to put their health and well-being last on
their priority list. Do family, career, and/or the business of the
day come before your WLS needs? Sacrifice and long hours at
work are rewarded in American society, which makes it easy
to neglect yourself.

After WLS, you will benefit from a change in priorities. Is
your health number one? Putting your health goals first
ensures that you will achieve them. When you practice putting your health first, and schedule everything else around it,
you will eventually find that doing so comes quite naturally.

Action for the day:

Today, evaluate whether you are putting your health first or
whether you are putting other things before your health.
Recommit to your health.

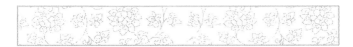

Keep head hunger in perspective.

Is your mind convinced it needs chocolate, chips, fries, ice cream, or some other comfort food? Of course, you know you don't really need those foods. You can look at your "head hunger" as a psychological call for comfort. Maybe you are feeling depressed, anxious, or bored. Do you want to cover up or soothe your feelings with food? How else can you cope with your uncomfortable feelings?

When hunger takes hold, keep your mind distracted from food and your hands busy. In your journal, write down what you want to accomplish as a thinner and healthier person and the type of life you want to live. Then, use your vision of the new you to put your head hunger in the proper perspective. You don't have to let head hunger rule your behavior.

Action for today:

Make a list of five activities that can be alternatives to stress eating. When the next urge to graze comes along, you'll be prepared.

Strive for balance.

To be truly happy, you need to balance all aspects of your life: mental, physical, spiritual, and emotional. If any one aspect is "off," you will feel out of sorts in all aspects. When you are tired physically, is your thinking as sharp? If your thinking is flawed, do your emotions become oppressive?

When your thinking is clear, you can more easily handle stress and your spirit is much happier. Balance is a critical component of your new life. Balance will help you maintain your weight loss.

Action for the day:

In your journal, make a heading for each aspect of your life: mental, physical, spiritual, and emotional. Under each aspect, how can you create more balance in your life? List three things you can do to move into balance...and then do them.

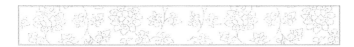

Don't let the hard work bother you.

Many people who have WLS are surprised at the amount of work the WLS lifestyle can require. Some people resent having to watch what they eat. They mistakenly believed prior to surgery that the procedure would take care of their food problem. A few misguided surgeons even tell their patients they are "cured."

The truth is that a healthy, rewarding life is hard work. But you decide whether it's worth it. Most thin people we know have to work at staying that way. They have to be self-disciplined, even when they don't want to be. Successful people we see, who are living their dreams, usually have worked very hard to get where they are. Hard work is a tool for you to use to get what you want in life. It is an opportunity. Take advantage of it.

Action for the day:

Think about one aspect of your WLS lifestyle you dislike. Now, visualize the REASON that aspect is necessary. Once you connect a difficult action with its positive goal, it becomes a bit less unsavory.

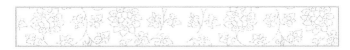

Learn to comfort yourself.

The longing for someone to share your burden can be worse than head hunger. But you will not always be able to get in touch with your support system. So, you will benefit from learning to comfort and support yourself.

Can you treat yourself to an afternoon of reading alone? How about going to a yoga class or getting a pedicure? There are so many ways to comfort yourself. Find what works for you.

Action for the day:

What feels really comforting to you (that isn't unhealthy)? Make a list to refer to when you are disconnected or lonely.

June

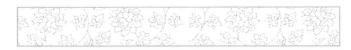

Happiness is not perfection.

Do you think that for you to be happy, everything in your life has to be just so? Happiness is a strange thing. It's not synonymous with perfection. In fact, some of the happiest people alive are neither wealthy…nor thin.

Happiness involves overlooking imperfections, laughing at mistakes, and making a lot of lemonade from lemons. It is the attitude you adopt even in the face of problems.

Action for the day:

Today, respond to your life with happiness. Wear your rose-colored glasses all day.

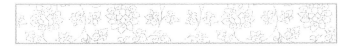

Enjoy your freedom.

After WLS, you continue day by day to cast off the chains that have bound you for so long. Each day you breathe better, move better, and feel better. You are free to enjoy not only your own life, but the lives of your family and friends as well.

Finally, you can play with your children outside. You can walk longer with your spouse or friends. You can say "yes" to invitations because you have the energy to endure the events, and you want to show off (just a little). Your family is excited to go on vacations that involve bathing suits and walking in the woods. And you equally share in the excitement of new places and new sites. Freedom from your weight is a wonderful feeling.

Action for the day:

What have you avoided doing in the past that you can do now? Today, take steps to do something that celebrates your new-found freedom.

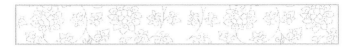

Wear clothes that fit.

For some people who have had WLS, buying clothes that fit correctly is a challenge. First, you may not see yourself as you really are; you may still have a "fat" brain—even if your body has slimmed down. And second, you may still be drawn to baggy clothes, thinking they will hide your physical flaws.

It may be time to rethink your fashion choices. Maybe something more form fitting will flatter you now. Maybe you still feel fat, but in reality you look fit and healthy.

Action for the day:

If you feel completely out of your element at the clothing store, or if you can't seem to let go of your baggy clothes, go shopping with a friend and let him or her dress you. Even if you don't buy, at least you'll start to see the possibilities.

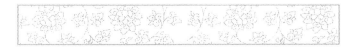

Be like Ferdinand.

Remember Ferdinand the Bull? He was a mild-mannered bull in a children's book, who liked to "sit just quietly" and smell the flowers. But Ferdinand was captured and taken to a bull fight. He was led out into the arena so the matador could fight him and stick him with his sword.

But Ferdinand chose not to fight. He just sat down and enjoyed the fragrance of flowers in the air. He refused to let the negative actions of others affect him.

Action for the day:

Today, if someone invites you to enter into an unpleasant conversation or a fight, choose to "sit just quietly," and don't let them push your buttons. You can be at peace when you know who you are and what you want—no matter what the rest of the world is doing.

June 5

Find what works for you.

Having WLS meant changing EVERYTHING about your life, and at first, it was a challenge learning how to take care of yourself. Then, perhaps, you entered a honeymoon phase. You knew what to do. You were feeling good, getting slimmer, and loving life. This phase is wonderful, and it lasts a long time for some people. For others, hunger returns more quickly. Living this new life gets harder and old habits return.

What will you do when you see old habits creeping back in? When you feel like you're slipping back, seek out and listen to the advice of others. Find out what works for them. But, then find what works for you. You know best what you will be willing to do long term. Summon the courage to take that knowledge and build a successful post-WLS life.

Action for the day:

Have you thought about how you'll handle the post-honeymoon phase? Today, in your journal, explore your options and identify the people you will turn to for advice. What might work for you?

June 6

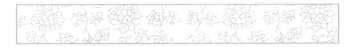

Track your lab work.

Don't assume that just because your lab work shows results in the normal range that you are okay. Be aware that for most people, shortages will not show up immediately. A downward trend in a lab value can still be in the normal range so that you don't even realize you are slipping.

When your surgeon or general practitioner says your lab values are fine, that isn't enough. Ask for a copy of your lab results and check them yourself. You are responsible for your well being and have the most to lose if there is an undetected problem.

Action for the day:

Make a chart or spreadsheet that lists out all the lab work you need to have done periodically and record your lab results each time you get tested. Check to make sure you are not in a downward trend that could lead to a deficiency.

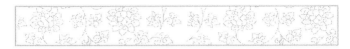

Be sugar free.

Sugar is addictive. No matter how much you want that not to be true, it is true. Most WLS patients, especially gastric bypass patients, avoid sugar after surgery, at least for awhile. But when they go back, they have trouble limiting themselves, just like in the old days before surgery.

The best gift you can give yourself is to never go back to eating sugar. If you already have gone back to it, and you can't seem to stop, try to come to terms with the idea that sugar is an addictive substance, and open yourself to the possibility of abstaining completely.

Action for the day:

If you are in the grips of sugar, read a book on the topic of either sugar addiction or food addiction. Begin to educate yourself about how to get off sugar and develop a plan to get it out of your life. You won't regret it.

Learn the difference between criticism and sharing your feelings.

It's easy to slip into judging others. In fact, it's human nature. But, when judging others turns into criticism, you can harm your relationships and become a negative influence. Did criticism ever help you? Probably not.

When someone's behavior affects you negatively, instead of criticizing them, the healthiest thing you can do is share with them how their behavior affects you—as kindly as possible. For example, you can say, "When you eat a huge bowl of ice cream day after day, I feel so anxious and fearful. I am afraid your unhealthy food choices will make you sick, and the thought of losing you breaks my heart."

Action for the day:

Pay attention to your thoughts and words today. Try to share your feelings about things that affect you without criticizing.

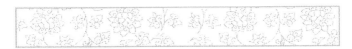

Ignore your impulse for instant gratification.

The need to feel good, or to relieve anxiety, or to entertain yourself is so compelling at times that, at first, giving in to it brings relief. Later, however, regret comes.

The pursuit of instant gratification undermines a healthy WLS lifestyle. Instead of trying to feel good in the moment, consider learning to tolerate some discomfort, so that you can experience the long-term satisfaction you really desire.

Action for the day:

Spend today noticing when you choose instant gratification over long-term satisfaction. In your journal, write about your self-discoveries. Do you have room for improvement?

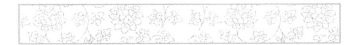

Empathize with others who suffer, but take care of yourself.

People may envy you now. They see you shrinking "effortlessly" while they struggle. Before, you were targeted for being oversized, now you are targeted for doing something about it.

When others look at you with envy, be sympathetic to their suffering, because you have been there. But don't entertain guilt or discount your effort with regard to WLS. Some people sabotage themselves when they feel their success is painful for others, but hurting yourself will not fix someone else. Learn to tolerate your success.

Action for the day:

Do you feel guilty or embarrassed about your success? In your journal, explore how it feels to be smaller when some of those around you are not.

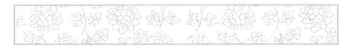

Listen to your body.

Are you sleep deprived? Do you wait until you're too hungry to eat? Being too tired or too hungry are great setups for disaster. Both situations can cause a person to eat more than they need.

It's one thing to have an occasional late night or to work through lunch every once in a while. But if this becomes the norm, consider bringing some balance into your life. Neglecting your body's needs will ultimately sabotage your WLS lifestyle.

Action for the day:

Live today with balance. Eat when you are hungry (but not too hungry), rest if you need it...pay attention to your body's needs.

Free yourself with mental and spiritual health.

After WLS the body will recover, but the true healing comes when your mind and soul are healed. You must examine how you got to the point of needing WLS, and address those issues before you can truly be free.

How do you "feed" your soul? What other ways can you relieve your stress? Have you let go of your shame? In short…are your mind and spirit healing along with your body?

Action for the day:

Spend five minutes today quietly contemplating your mental and spiritual condition. Will they support WLS success? Now that your body is healing, explore how you can pursue the healing of your mind and spirit.

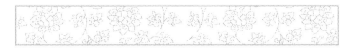

Take a dose of humility along with your success.

Have you ever had someone tell you how they think you should live? Did you feel annoyed...even hurt? As you transform, your success can become a point of pride for you. But avoid the temptation to act as if you know it all, as if you know how others should lose weight, as if you are better than people who are struggling.

You can be satisfied with your progress and know it was the right path for you. But each person must choose their own destiny and come to their own decision. Remember how you felt when people tried to tell you what to do. Be gracious and compassionate with people, keeping your well-meaning opinions to yourself when they are not solicited.

Action for the day:

Practice humility today. Start by thinking of a time when someone practiced humility toward you.

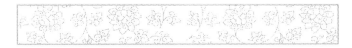

Act, don't react.

Are you reacting to challenging situations or are you taking
deliberate action? Reaction is what your gut tells you to do in
the moment. It is spontaneous and often not the healthiest
response.

But when you take deliberate action in a situation, you ensure
that your response is more effective. You take a mental step
back from the challenging situation and evaluate what is
happening first. Second, you determine what will likely
happen in response to your actions. You can ask yourself,
"What is the ultimate outcome I want in this situation?"
Think things through, and then, rather than react, perform a
deliberate action.

Action for the day:

Take time to deliberate on your actions today instead of
reacting spontaneously. Practice thinking things through
before you act.

Get back to basics.

Sometimes life gets complicated. You are busy. Maybe you are going through a big change, like a move. Or maybe you're getting over an illness that kept you from eating your usual fare. Somehow, when you get a bit off-track, it can be hard to see your way back. The best solution is to get back to basics.

Drink at least 64 oz. of water. Have three to five appropriately -sized meals. Chew slowly and thoroughly. Eat protein first, then veggies, and finally, if you have room, a small amount of complex carbs. Take your vitamins and supplements. Move your body (even if it's just doing a little housework or taking the stairs instead of the elevator).

Action for the day:

Make today a "back to basics" day.

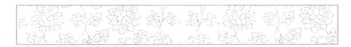

Use your gifts.

We all have wonderful, unique talents, and it would be a loss not to use them for a greater good. The truth is that the world needs you to use your gifts to bless others.

Through WLS, you have been reborn into this life; let that rebirth have a great purpose. Will you inspire someone? Will you make the world a better place? Will you pursue a life-long dream? Many opportunities exist to produce a worthy product from the gifts you have been given. Use those opportunities with gratitude and joy.

Action for the day:

In your journal, explore your gifts. What will you do with them? Take an action today that involves using one of your gifts.

Be conscious today.

Sometimes people go through life performing their tasks
without really thinking about them. It's easy to get so caught
up in things that you don't pay attention to what's behind
what you're doing.

Overeating can be an unconscious act. It is possible to think
back on your day and realize you have been grazing a lot or
that you ate the donut that was offered to you without even
blinking. To make the lifestyle changes required of a WLS
patient, you must learn to be present and aware as you go
through your day.

Action for the day:

Today, practice being conscious. With every action you take,
pause first and ask yourself, "What am I doing and why?" In
your journal, write about your discoveries.

Avoid temptation.

If a cookie is sitting on your counter at home, you are more likely to eat it than if the cookie is in your pantry (or in the store). Despite the simplicity of this idea, many WLS patients keep tempting foods in plain sight and try to convince themselves they won't eat it—but then they do.

If you really want to have some success at losing or maintaining, then remove temptation from your life as much as possible. You don't have absolute control of your environment, but you are not helpless, either.

Action for the day:

Look through your home and office today. What temptations can you get rid of? With whom should you set limits so that you are not constantly bombarded with tempting foods?

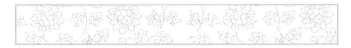

Slow down.

Life can get hectic. Sometimes things are out of your control and you just have to do the best you can. Other times things are stresses you bring upon yourself. Your new life after WLS needs to be based on balance and a commitment to take care of yourself like never before. Too much stress can increase your appetite. Is that what you really want?

A very wise person once prayed, "Lord, grant me the strength to accept the things I cannot change, the courage to change the things I can, and the wisdom to know the difference." Amen to that.

Action for the day:

Evaluate your schedule. Is there anything you can cancel? Is there someone you can ask to help? Be brave today and take control of your schedule based on your long-term health goals.

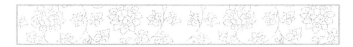

Make that big decision.

A decision to change your life is a big step, not easily taken.
It is something you need to take time to consider. A big
decision needs to be made in a moment of true consciousness,
when you are able to see clearly what you are doing, and
what the outcome of your actions will be. In that moment,
you can acknowledge where you are and decide to change
your course.

If deep down you know you need to make a big decision, you
can start the process. Change can be scary, but if you make
your decision as an outgrowth of being in touch with yourself
and your true needs, you won't go wrong. Have courage.

Action for the day:

In your journal, write about a decision you need to make.
Spend some time thinking about your decision and defining
it. Then, MAKE IT.

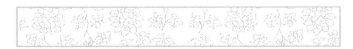

Ignore your "don't wannas."

Do you ever wake up and think, "I don't wanna follow my regimen today." When you have that feeling, instead of dwelling on it, focus your thoughts on your next right action. Tell yourself, "I can get up and take my vitamins." Then do it.

Each time you feel doubt or dread, switch your focus to what is in front of you. You can do this next thing—even if you can't follow your program all day. As you go through your day, though, keep doing the next right thing. You'll be thrilled with how much you get done.

Action for the day:

Don't entertain your feelings of dread or hopelessness today. Focus on what is possible in the moment—not on what you have coming up later on.

Look within.

It is healthy to look within. To find peace and serenity, you must put pride and fear aside and take an honest look at yourself.

Find the courage and resolve to discover yourself. Find out what makes you tick. Find out how you sabotage yourself and why. Learn what really motivates you. Seeking fixes and answers outside of yourself can only take you so far. To achieve fulfillment, you must look within.

Action for the day:

Spend five minutes today looking within. Sit quietly and breathe deeply. Ask yourself, "What is it that I need to find and acknowledge within myself to become healthy?"

Care for your body.

After all your body has been through, it still carries you and tries to keep you healthy. You can care for this incredible machine by slowing down your day, taking time to eat, remembering to chew completely and hydrating properly.

But most importantly, you need to take time to think, time to clear your head of all the many distractions of the day, time to evaluate your goals and whether or not you are meeting them, time to breathe and enjoy your new, healthier self.

Action for the day:

Make time today to care for your incredible body.

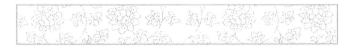

Eat anything you want, whenever you want, at your peril.

Eating with free abandon is not freedom for people who struggle with compulsive eating. Grazing all day means you have no structure to your eating. And unstructured eating can quickly lead to eating unhealthy foods in unhealthy portions.

Ironically, when you add some structure to your eating by making a food plan for the day, an amazing sense of freedom can set in. When you set boundaries for your food, it may be difficult for a time, but eventually freedom will come.

Action for the day:

Make a food plan today. Write it down and refer to it often. Give yourself the gift of one day of freedom from overeating.

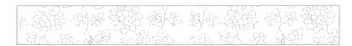

Don't let the scale make you crazy.

Many people use the scale to determine how they should feel about themselves on a given day. If it is frozen or moving up, they get a strong urge to throw in the towel and eat, eat, eat. But paying such close attention to the scale and making self-judgments based on its movements is not motivating. You haven't gone through WLS to be uncomfortable and to feel badly about yourself.

Yes, you need to check your weight consistently, but you do not have to check it daily. And you can work on the self talk you use when you do weigh yourself. If the scale makes you crazy, then you know what you need to work on. You can work on changing how you think about the scale and how you treat yourself as a result of weighing.

Action for the day:

In your journal, write about your feelings when you weigh yourself. Are you at peace with weighing? Take some time to sort out what you can do to bring some sanity into your relationship with your scale.

Explore new territory.

Getting on a bicycle for the first time may be scary for you. Buying your first pair of non-stretch pants may seem impossible. Maybe you're terrified with the thought of dating. But, shaping the new life you want will involve getting out of your comfort zone. It will mean trying something different.

Expect to be uncomfortable, but also expect to feel proud and thrilled with each and every success. You are creating the life you've always wanted.

Action for the day:

Is there something you want to do that feels too frightening? Take a step today toward that goal. Find a buddy if you need to, but take action.

Find healthy ways to deal with emotions.

Do you deal with your feelings now the same as you did before weight loss surgery? Most WLS patients were emotional eaters before their surgery. Food probably was your comfort.

But, you can choose to react differently to strong emotions today, rather than being a victim of them. First, find the willingness to try new things in response to your feelings. Then, experiment. It may take awhile to find other ways to relieve your emotional stress. Some people process their feelings by writing in a journal, others take up yoga. There are myriad things you can try.

Action for the day:

In your journal, make a written plan for times when you find yourself feeling overwhelmed with emotion.

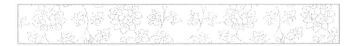

Maintain your motivation.

What sparks your inner fire and drives you to act? One of
the hardest things to maintain after weight loss surgery is
motivation. A honeymoon period keeps many WLS patients
on track for the first six months to two years, but eventually
almost everyone loses their momentum—at least sometimes.

One tool you can have at the ready is knowing what
motivates you. Something empowered you to take control of
your health. Look along that path for clues.

Action for the day:

In your journal, list the times in your life when you felt
empowered and took brave action. Look for clues about what
motivated you in those moments. How can you use this
knowledge about yourself to stay on a healthy path now?

Nurture your soul.

Your mind races constantly with all the many things you need to do. Yet even in the midst of all your obligations, you must take time to nurture your soul.

A wonderful way to get centered—and to get exercise as a bonus—is yoga. Yoga will increase your flexibility, muscle tone, and mental focus. Breathing techniques help to slow down your body and mind. You learn to relax at a very deep level. You also learn to relate to your body in a new and empowering way.

Action for the day:

Find out if there is a yoga class you can add to your life. The effort will be well worth it.

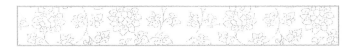

Use your support network.

Sometimes the most effective way to feel better is to get help with a problem, rather than falling into self pity. When you connect with another WLS patient, you can support each other through the ups and downs after surgery. Keep in mind that asking for help can be just as supportive as helping another. You can call for help when your resolve is weak and know you will be understood. Asking for help is strength, although many people feel like they are going to bother someone or they are afraid.

The more you ask for help, the easier it becomes to call on your support system. Before you know it, this system will become a vital part of your life.

Action for the day:

Remaining part of a support network is still important, no matter how far out from surgery you get. Today, check on a fellow WLS patient to see how he or she is doing.

July

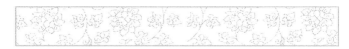

Admit WLS isn't enough.

Sometimes in the early days after WLS, people are in a honeymoon phase. No matter how educated you are about WLS and its potential pitfalls, during the honeymoon phase you will think you are immune from those pitfalls. You will refuse to believe it's possible to go back to where you were before surgery. But it's possible.

There comes a time for most obesity survivors when WLS isn't enough. Your pouch may not be enough to keep you from losing or maintaining your weight loss. You may hit a wall. Old behaviors may creep back in. Trigger foods may become easier to tolerate. You may have a crisis that leads you to emotional eating and your healed pouch will tolerate your comfort foods.

Action for the day:

Think about how your longer term WLS recovery will be. What tools can you have in place to help you respond when your surgery alone isn't enough anymore?

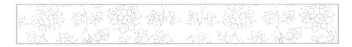

Fill your life with goals.

When you get close to your weight goal, you become more focused on it. You think about it constantly. Will it be tomorrow? In three days? Next week? Every time you eat you may think, "Maybe if I eat a little less, I can get to my goal sooner," or, "What if I walk twice a day for just this week?" Or, maybe you think, "After I reach my goal I can relax, right?"

You may think that once you reach goal you are done. But you will need to remain ever-vigilant caring for your pouch, which is still your most valuable tool. You also will need to see beyond weight loss to the other things in life that make it worth living. Learn something new. Set a goal to meet a different kind of challenge. Fill your life with more goals than just reaching your goal weight, and see how full your life can be.

Action for the day:

Choose one of your goals and make progress on it today.

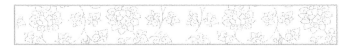

Don't wait.

Today is all you have. This moment is what's real. Who knows what the next moment, or tomorrow, will bring? So ask yourself, "What can I accomplish today?"

This is your time to create the life you want. Procrastination gains you nothing. In fact, it robs you of the better life you desire. When faced with an action, have you said, "I'll do that when I'm thinner"? You don't have to wait. You can get busy today and make headway toward your goals.

Action for the day:

Do three things you have been putting off.

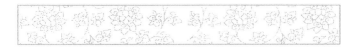

Let go of old ideas.

Some weight loss surgery patients are afraid to eat when they are told to progress from pureed to solid food—and they restrict what they eat. Others start sneaking foods they miss early on, and suffer the physical consequences.

WLS does not remove misguided ideas about food and eating. It only makes your stomach smaller and sometimes introduces a malabsorptive component. What you think about food and how you eat is your job to evaluate and modify. You might need some help from a nutritionist, coach, or therapist. The "new you" wants to take responsibility for practicing a new way of thinking and a new way of approaching food. Do you have a sane approach to eating and food that is based on your new physical and emotional needs?

Action for the day:

Take a few minutes today to consider how you think about eating and food. Are your ideas about these things going to serve you well now?

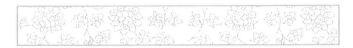

Put first things first.

Do you sometimes eat what you like best first, knowing you have limited space in your stomach? Do you sometimes do volunteer work, socialize, watch an old movie, or shop for clothes instead of doing your exercise or taking the time to prepare healthy meals?

Enjoy your food, see your friends, volunteer, and do all of the other wonderful activities you enjoy, but put your health first. The WLS lifestyle is rigorous, and your health needs must come first if you are to overcome obesity once and for all.

Action for the day:

Put first things first today. Eat your dense protein before your brown rice and veggies. Exercise before you read your mystery novel. Cut up fresh veggies you can eat for the next few days before you check your email.

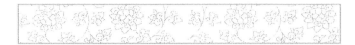

Learn to recognize true friends.

A true friend may be hard to recognize at first. Many obese
people have had inferiority issues their entire lives, and hence
sometimes let others treat them in ways that are negative,
even abusive. Abusive, unkind people are like unsightly weeds
in our gardens.

A true friend builds you up, makes you stronger, and supports
your healthy growth. True friends are like water on a thirsty
flower bed. They feed your soul.

Action for the day:

Spend some time thinking about your friends today. Do
they support your healthy growth? It may be time to "pluck
some weeds."

Don't overreact to overeating.

So, you've made a small blunder in your diet. Treat it as a
small blunder.

When you make a misstep, do not then give in to the
temptation to throw in the towel altogether. Just say, "Oops,"
and then do the next right thing. The mistake is not as important as what you do in response to it. Chalk up the incident to
being human, forgive yourself, and jump right back on track.

Action for the day:

Whenever you find yourself straying from your WLS lifestyle,
pause and ask yourself, "What is the next right thing to do?"
Then, do it.

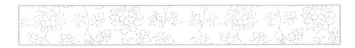

Stand up.

Standing up for yourself and being who you are can be very
hard. But you do not have to give in to the pressures of life.
You can remain true to yourself. Yes, it is often easier to fall
into line with the rest of society. But the long-term results can
be devastating, especially when it comes to food. So many
temptations exist that are unhealthy; you just can't afford to
indulge all the time.

Do you want to be a mindless automaton in the machine
of life? Or do you want to take control of that machine?
After WLS, following in the way of the world can mean
disaster. Shaping your new reality to meet your needs will
lead to success.

Action for the day:

Walk your own path today. The one that will lead you to the
great health and well-being for which you have longed.

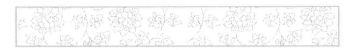

Grocery shop strategically.

Have you ever noticed that when you go to the grocery store hungry you come home with a lot of junk and food you don't normally eat? Or that when you go to the grocery store alone you are more likely to buy a food you want to sneak eat? Do you buy foods you don't really need when you skip making a shopping list?

If grocery stores are hard for you, be willing to develop a strategy for success. For example, shop after dinner. Or bring a WLS friend with you to be an accountability partner. If you have to, have someone shop for you during difficult times.

Action for the day:

Do you need a better grocery-shopping strategy? If so, today come up with a plan to try, and enlist the support you need.

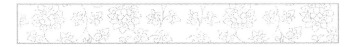

Make friends with your scale.

At first, after surgery, the scale is fun. The weight is dropping and you feel good. Over time, though, for some WLS patients, old eating patterns can creep back in, and it becomes harder to want to weigh yourself.

Fear of the scale sets in for some people, and avoidance takes over. But, one of the keys to long-term success is to know how much you weigh. Checking your weight every week is a great way to stay out of denial. If you start to gain, you can do something about it before the problem gets out of control.

Action for the day:

Make a weight chart and start tracking your weight. If you go up more than a couple of pounds, take action to bring your weight back down again.

Swim.

You wait at water's edge as your ship of dreams sails close to
the horizon, and you wish it would come to shore. Your
dreams are afloat, but they will not come to you. To realize
your dreams, you must be willing to work for them—
to "swim out" to them.

It's time to jump into the water and chase your ship. You are
sleeker and faster now. You are stronger and have more
endurance. You can reach that ship, pull yourself up over the
railing, and declare yourself the captain of your life.

Action for the day:

In your journal, write down one or more of your life-long
dreams. Have you stuck a toe in the water yet? If not, get
started. You have a long way to swim, but you have already
come a long way. You can do it.

Take care of yourself.

You probably don't schedule your day like this: 9 o'clock: eat breakfast, 10 o'clock: get your hair cut, 11 o'clock: have a crisis, 12 o'clock: go to the dentist. The crisis arrives uninvited and forces you to change your life around it. *Webster's* defines a crisis as a "turning point in the course of anything." Some crises are worse than others, yet they all are turning points.

Just breathe. A clear head will get you through your crisis. Concentrate on your WLS plan to minimize the impact, and take good care of yourself.

Action for the day:

How do you handle crises? In your journal, describe the types of crises that have driven you to overeat or to be self-destructive in the past. Then, make a plan you can use when faced with a crisis. List out exactly what you will do to take care of yourself.

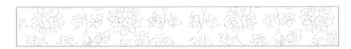

Express yourself.

Throughout your life, you have used food to deal with your emotions. Years spent "stuffing" your feelings with food have probably diminished your ability to express yourself in other ways—like crying.

Tears, for most, serve as a welcome release in a crisis. Perhaps you want to cry, but seem to have forgotten how. You don't know what to do with the pain now that you can't overeat.

Action for the day:

Today, practice releasing any negative emotions in a healthy way. If crying won't work, try hitting something. Yell into a pillow, call a friend (don't yell at your friend, though), exercise a bit. Find what works for you.

Do some soul searching.

What makes you feel alive? Is it the feeling of contributing something important to the world? Is it love of children or family or pets? Is it spiritual fulfillment?

Often what people think is important is what they were taught by their parents. While your parents may have instilled in you good morals and values, what was important to them may be infinitely different from what is important to you. You must decide what you value for yourself. What truly matters in your life? Are your priorities arranged according to what matters to you?

Action for the day:

In your journal, write about the things in life that are really important to you. Then, explore how you can organize your life to make it reflect what truly matters to you.

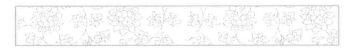

Contribute to the discussion.

Have you been shy about stating your opinion? Have you worried that what you say will not be taken seriously? Maybe you've experienced obesity discrimination, which has left you uncomfortable with calling attention to yourself for fear of being judged or ridiculed.

It's time to reframe your view of yourself. You have an important perspective to contribute. Don't worry about whether your idea is the best; it just may be the seed that sparks a great revelation.

Action for the day:

Your ideas will never be used if you do not find the courage to speak them. Share your thoughts with someone today.

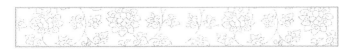

Keep food in a healthy perspective.

To be successful after WLS, it's best to get your comfort from things other than food. Comfort can come from hugs, from wrapping in a warm blanket, from turning to a friend, from journaling your thoughts, and from keeping your hands busy.

Try to think of food as nourishment for your body, and look for new things to nourish your soul. Food is a necessary part of our day, but not the whole of it.

Action for the day:

Are you thinking too much about food? Today, when you notice yourself thinking about food (other than at meal time), practice changing your focus.

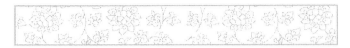

Make an effort.

If a musically inexperienced person sat down at a piano
without ever having read a note, her first attempt would
sound awful. Yet with education and practice, eventually she
would play a pleasing piece.

What will make an inexperienced musician successful is a
willingness to practice and to tolerate the discomfort of
making mistakes. That attitude is what will make you
successful with weight loss surgery.

Action for the day:

Are you struggling with maintaining a healthy lifestyle?
All you can do is try. If you don't try, you'll never improve.
So today, try.

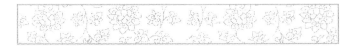

Care for the child in you today.

When you are taking care of a child, your priority is to give them a safe, healthy, and loving environment.

People who are, or have been, obese can sometimes put their own needs aside. You deserve the same special environment any child does. You are precious, too.

Action for the day:

Is your environment reflective of someone who takes special care of a loved one (themselves)? Today, think about how you parent yourself.

Distract yourself.

Eating out of boredom or to relieve anxiety can be a big problem for WLS patients. To avoid grazing for these reasons, you simply need to distract yourself. Distracting yourself means finding something to do or think about that is absorbing enough to put food out of your thoughts for awhile.

Other than food, what do you enjoy doing? Watching a movie? Calling a friend? Taking a walk? Organizing a closet?

Action for the day:

In your journal, make a list of distractions that seem fun, interesting, and/or consuming for you. Post your list on the refrigerator and read it whenever you feel like grazing. Pick one or two distractions and give them a try.

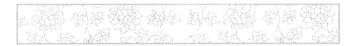

Do your work.

Sometimes people who have WLS are disappointed when
they realize that to have a lasting recovery, they will have to
work at it. Work, for them, has purely negative connotations.
But, if you are doing what you love, work becomes worthwhile, even enjoyable. But how do you learn to love the work
required of WLS patients?

Understand the long-term benefits of the work you are doing.
Will having more energy (because you've taken your vitamins)
give you the "oomph" you need to take on that extra project
that gets you a raise? Does a fit and healthy body make you
more confident finding a mate? WLS patients must accept
that life is work for everyone. You are not exempt, but your
attitude will make all the difference.

Action for the day:

Today, in your journal, make a list of some of the reasons you
want to have lasting success with WLS.

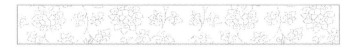

Avoid Avoidance.

It's common for people to avoid things they think will be
unpleasant. But what is the cost? You want to quit your job,
but you're afraid to tell your boss. So, you stay at a job that
makes you unhappy. Every time you think about telling him
or her, you feel anxious. And in between feeling trapped on
the job and anxious, you feel miserable. That level of anxiety
and stress is a set-up for making poor food choices.

When you take care of something unpleasant immediately,
you spare yourself a lot of hardship. The pain is short-lived,
and you can get on with your life.

Action for the day:

Have you been avoiding something you need to do? Take care
of it today. Free yourself from the anxiety and dread.

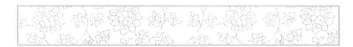

Do something differently.

WLS patients come to understand their surgery is no cure for
obesity. In fact, it is very common for patients to regain some
of their weight. A small weight regain may be normal, but
huge gains usually can be avoided with education, effort, and
careful attention to living a new, healthy WLS lifestyle.

The bottom line for most is that if you don't change what
you've always done, you're going to keep getting what you've
always gotten—even after weight loss surgery.

Action for the day:

Begin establishing a new habit that is positive today. Do
SOMETHING differently.

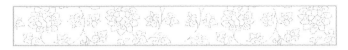

Play.

The older you get, the more important it is for you to not act your age. As you lose weight, you feel lighter than you have in years. Your body moves easily and you may realize you have the urge to play, to frolic. Give in. When your children beg you to come outside and play with them—do it. You can joyously jump into the pile of leaves you've raked. You can unashamedly make a snow angel and get up without help.

Rejoicing in your newfound youth, you reawaken your inner child. This awakening releases your soul and lets it soar. You are limited only by yourself and your inhibitions. Now is your time to play like you haven't in a long, long time.

Action for the day:

You guessed it. Play.

Don't keep it a secret.

You have been given a great gift with WLS—the opportunity
to be free of obesity. Even though the WLS lifestyle can
require a lot of effort, most WLS patients would not trade
their opportunity for anything. WLS is a hopeful process,
with many rewards.

In addition to keeping an attitude of gratitude, be sure to pass
along your discovery. Be the light in someone's life who needs
the kind of hope you now have.

Action for the day:

How can you pass along an opportunity for a better life to
someone else in need? Meditate on that today, and come up
with an action you can take.

Discover who you are.

Do you worry about what other people think of you? You might find more peace in this world if you become more concerned about what YOU think of you. Are you always trying to be someone you are not in order to please someone else?

You will not reach your full potential if you are putting all your energy into becoming what the world wants you to become. When you are true to yourself, you will attract friends who like you for who you really are.

Action for the day:

In your journal, write a description of yourself as you truly want to be. Read it often.

Take advantage of wisdom.

If only people were born with all the wisdom they would need to get through life. Everything would be so much easier that way.

The journey to wisdom is a long and painful process littered with regrets and mistakes. But each mistake is a learning experience that adds to your wisdom. And the road ahead is always brighter, because you have learned, and will continue to learn, from your mistakes.

Action for the day:

Meditate on wisdom today. Are you using this powerful and hard-earned tool? When you are faced with a challenge, ask yourself, "What is the wise thing for me to do?"

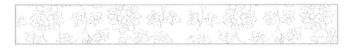

Be optimistic.

The biggest reason for success is attitude. If you believe you will succeed, you are much more likely to. A successful person is someone who refuses to give up even after several failures, believing that the next attempt will finally work.

Even if the odds are against you, the belief that anything is possible if you work hard enough will get you closer to your goal than believing the opposite.

Action for the day:

Today, tell yourself you will not fail. (Look in the mirror and say it out loud.) Take a bold action to move yourself toward your goal.

Take time for yourself today.

Even though it may be raining, the dog is barking, your
spouse or partner is moody, your boss is on a rampage, or it
feels like the world is falling in on you, take a moment to do
something for yourself.

Your mental health rests on taking time for yourself, affirming
your spirit, and stopping the chaos in its tracks if only for a
few moments. Let the rest of the world wait; you have
something important to do—take care of you. This act of
self-affirmation can be as simple as having a cup of tea in a
stolen moment of the afternoon or five minutes of reading a
fascinating article while locked in the bathroom. It can be a
few extra minutes in a warm shower, a brisk walk, a good
stretch, or sitting cuddled with your child or spouse or kitty.

Action for the day:

No matter what is going on in your life today, take a few
moments to affirm yourself. Claim a little time for you.

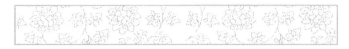

Strive for consistency.

Being consistent every day is tough. You may want to think that because you made healthy choices yesterday it's okay to slack off a bit today.

Consistency may seem boring or frustrating at first, but it becomes a very satisfying way of life once you get used to it. You learn you can trust yourself, and you begin to feel more grounded.

Action for the day:

If you were going to be more consistent with your WLS lifestyle, what would your life look like, ideally? In your journal, describe this lifestyle. Then live it for a few days. See how it feels to nurture yourself by being predictable.

Remember prayer.

If you are a person who longs for a connection to a higher power, you might want to consider prayer as a tool on your WLS journey. It's surprising how many people simply forget or don't take the time to pray.

Prayer can center you and help you gain perspective on your life. It can remind you of what is really important and what is not. Prayer is the practice of humility, of demonstrating that you do not know all the answers and that you are open to help. It is a hopeful act that can ease your worries and inform your actions.

Action for the day:

If you would like to feel a connection to your higher power, take a few minutes to pray today. If you are not comfortable with prayer, think about how you can nurture and develop your spirit.

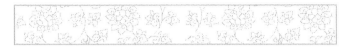

Surrender.

Are you still in the "food fight"? Do you continue to test your limits, eating beyond satisfaction or grazing? Are you spending your days planning to eat, eating, and regretting eating?

This is a vicious cycle that you can end. It's time to surrender. Time to admit that your way isn't working and to try someone else's plan. If you are unsure of what you need to be eating, make an appointment with a WLS-knowledgeable nutritionist. Surrender means you let go of the cycle, choosing instead to open yourself up to the guidelines of people who have a healthier perspective on eating.

Action for the day:

Think about your current relationship with food. Are you worried and obsessed, or are you at peace? Take an honest look, and if you are still fighting with food, it's time to negotiate a surrender. Make an appointment with a nutritionist and reach out to your support system.

August

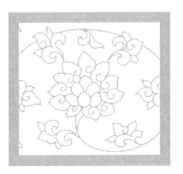

Break down your goals into "bite-sized" chunks.

To get to the top of Mt. Everest is a huge feat, even for experienced climbers. Even they take the mountain in small steps. They climb a certain distance, then rest.

Think about how you can use this approach in your own life. Over time, you can reach even your loftiest goals. Take it one step at a time.

Action for the day:

Pick a task you've wanted to accomplish, but have been putting off. Today set a timer and work for 20 minutes. When the timer goes off, decide whether you will keep working for 20 minutes more or if you are done for the day. Either way, you have moved closer to your goal.

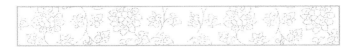

Invest in yourself.

Sometimes your WLS routine feels like drudgery. You don't feel like drinking another glass of water. You are too tired to exercise. You just don't want to have to think about what you're putting in your mouth.

Think of following your surgeon's or dietician's guidelines like putting money in the bank. Every investment in your new lifestyle will help build your "wealth of health" in the long run.

Action for the day:

Make an investment in your health today. Spend five minutes visualizing how you want to feel, look, and live in the long run.

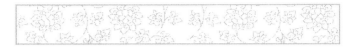

Ask for help.

It is estimated that 70 percent of weight loss surgery patients have an eating disorder, also known as a food addiction. The number one reason most people avoid seeking help for food addiction is they don't believe they can stop their negative eating behaviors. They have such a track record of failure with weight loss and weight control that they feel absolutely hopeless.

The truth is people recover from food addiction all the time. You can, too. Consider asking for help.

Action for the day:

Do you struggle with a food addiction? If you are not sure, do some online research today. If you do have a food addiction, research online to find out what kinds of help are available to you.

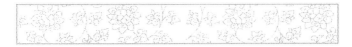

Set your angel free.

When you decided to have weight loss surgery, were you longing to set free something inside you? Obesity had hidden your true self from view. You longed to reveal the inner you. So, each day WLS has chipped away at your exterior.

Michelangelo said, "I saw the angel in the stone and carved until I set him free." Yet at the end of his first day, the rock still looked like…a rock. Only slowly did it become the beautiful creation that was locked within. As you lose weight, you will change many times; you will wake up mornings and not recognize the thinner face that has replaced the rounded one. In time, with consistency, effort, and a firm vision, you will release your angel within.

Action for the day:

Today, set aside a few quiet moments and visualize the inner you—your inner angel. In your mind, embrace that vision, talk to it, and plan together how your inner angel can help you remain steadfast.

Shield yourself from your triggers.

Are there trigger foods that get you every single time? All you have to do is smell them, or see them, and the next thing you know you're licking your fingers and savoring the lingering flavor. If you're like most WLS patients, though, you find that other than the fleeting moment of bliss you experience as you bite into the trigger food, you feel disappointed in yourself. And fear of completely losing control sets in. Why can't you resist that temptation?

It doesn't matter why. Food is tempting, and certain foods are nearly irresistible. So what can you do? Shield your senses from the most alluring foods. If you don't see it, and you can't smell it, you are much less likely to eat it. Create a safety zone in which you do not have to see, smell, and resist trigger foods all the time.

Action for the day:

Choose a trigger food that has been enticing you recently. Remove it from your house today. If you think this will be difficult for you, enlist the help of a trusted friend. Have him or her come over and help you get rid of the trigger food.

Hold your horses.

Eating out can be an enjoyable social event, and most WLS patients don't want to miss out. But do you have a plan for how you'll handle the appetizers? It's hard to resist that mouth-watering fare as others at your table dig in. While you may not want to eat too much, you also don't want to avoid the appetizer altogether if you will feel deprived.

If you tend to feel deprived and then overeat later on in private, go ahead and have a taste. To keep the amount you eat to a minimum, put off your taste until most of the appetizer is gone. Just reassure yourself you're going to have some soon, and enjoy the conversation.

Action for the day:

If you are in a restaurant today and are faced with the appetizer dilemma, delay as long as you can. This way, you'll have less time (and less food) to eat.

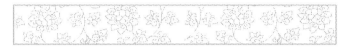

Stay focused.

Life is full of distractions. Your company is downsizing, your debt has become unmanageable, your basement has flooded again—the list is endless.

What is the one thing that would make all this worse? You know all too well. Being obese and ill. Certainly, life can hand us whoppers—challenges beyond what we feel we can handle—but most of your stresses are distractions from what is truly important. Most of them need to take second place to your health.

Action for the day:

Are you allowing life's distractions to interfere with living the lifestyle (physically, mentally, and spiritually) that will keep you healthy in the long run? In your journal, write a list of the distractions that are robbing you of the success you desire. Resolve not to let distractions steal your resolve.

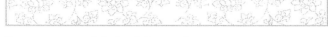

Designate a "default" meal.

There are times when you just want to eat the way you used to eat before surgery. It's hard to adjust to a new way of eating. And while sometimes it's pretty easy, sometimes it's not.

Find a meal that you can use as a "default" meal—the meal you always have when you are struggling. Find out what really tastes good and satisfies you, and is also good for you. Make this highly satisfying and healthy meal when you are having the most trouble. Serve it only on those occasions when you feel at wit's end. It will be your "ace in the hole."

Action for the day:

Make a list of the foods and meals you love that are also good for you. If you have trouble identifying these meals, keep a log of healthy meals you have eaten for a week or two, and rate each one on a scale of 1 to 10 (10 being the best). The next time you are having a particularly tough day, make one of the "10" meals.

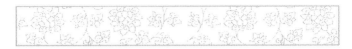

Make decisions based on facts, not feelings.

In 12-step programs there is a saying: "There are only two times to go to a 12-step meeting: when you want to go and when you don't want to go." How can you apply this philosophy to your WLS lifestyle? Do you think it is a good idea to base what you do (with exercise and food choices) on how you feel?

If you only do the right thing when you feel like it, how likely are you to lose your excess weight and keep it off for life?

Action for the day:

Today, do what supports your WLS success. For example, don't base your decision to exercise on whether or not you feel like it. Do it because you have planned to do it. No excuses.

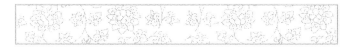

Rescue yourself.

Do you sometimes feel like you just want someone to come into your life and solve all your problems? A new relationship to make you happy, a new boss to replace the current micro-manager, a new neighbor who will go for a walk with you in the evenings.

You can choose to stay trapped in your disappointing situation. OR...you can change jobs, make new friends, or find a way to make exercise fun—even if you have to do it alone. You can refuse to slip into self pity, learn to be forgiving, or work on expressing your feelings in a healthy way.

Action for the day:

Today, think of ways you can rescue yourself.

Keep a short list.

It's okay to have grand goals and a long list of things you'd like to eventually accomplish in your lifetime. Just make sure you don't use that master list as your day-to-day list. Reading such a long, daunting list may prove to be so discouraging you'll convince yourself you'll never accomplish anything.

Better to make a short list that includes only a few goals at a time. Then work on your short list of goals for the day. You'll have plenty of time to get to the others on the master list. Each day brings with it the chance to accomplish more. Do it in manageable chunks, and you'll soon be pleasantly surprised at how fast you're checking items off.

Action for the day:

Review your "to-do" list to make sure it isn't overwhelming. Put your master list in a place where it won't be constantly visible, and vow to consult it only when you've completed your short list.

Find an honest friend.

You're bound to stumble every once in awhile. Everyone does. What people often need at those times is someone who will help nudge them back on track. This support person must be gentle, loving, and, perhaps more importantly, truthful.

Maybe you know someone who is always honest. Someone who can say, if need be, "I'm worried about you. I think your choice is hurting you." In other words, someone who is not afraid to challenge you, but who will not undermine you. Someone who can help you, but not enable you. Trust this person to pull you back to reality during times of difficulty.

Action for the day:

Think of one person in your life, whether it's a family member, a friend, or even a colleague, who can help you stay on track by being honest with you. Resolve to ask that person to confront you when you push your limits.

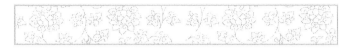

Be patient in your efforts.

Most people long for a quick fix to their eating problems. They don't want to have to work at it or wait for the much-delayed reward.

But, patience is what it takes—countless hours of trying various tools and finding out which ones work best. Then, you have to put in more hours practicing new behaviors. Shaping a new life that really works requires painstaking effort.

Action for the day:

Pay attention to your attitude about your WLS lifestyle today. Are you impatient or rebellious? Practice patience today. Trust the process.

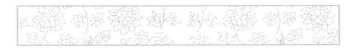

Be congruent.

Is there a difference between what you say you want and what you do? For example, do you say you want to maintain your weight, but then spend your afternoon snacking?

Being congruent involves aligning your desires with your actions. It's hard, and it is not a skill you can master overnight. Congruency is a worthy goal, however, and will greatly improve with practice.

Action for the day:

For today, practice being congruent. If you say you are tired and need to rest, don't go out dancing.

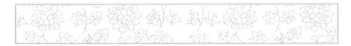

Remember to kihap.

In the martial art of Taekwondo, students are reminded to kihap, or "spirit yell," with every move. Most people may not know the term, but they've probably heard the strange, forceful burst of sound that martial artists emit when they kick or punch. It's not done just to sound like Bruce Lee. The real purpose is to focus all of your energy into that one kick or punch. It focuses your mind, and calls up all of your energy for that one task.

Obviously, you can't be going around your office or the local mall kihaping all day. But the lesson can be applied to your everyday life and tasks. Try focusing your full attention and energy on the task at hand.

Action for the day:

Reflect on recent times in which your mind has not stayed on task. With each new activity today, think of a simple statement—even something as simple as, "I am about to..." in order to focus your energy on the task at hand.

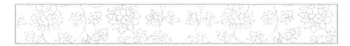

Develop calluses on your feelings.

Guitar players gradually develop hard calluses on their fingertips from pressing down on the narrow strings. Initially, playing can be painful and cause blisters or bleeding. But eventually, the calluses harden and enable the guitarist to play without discomfort.

As someone who has struggled with obesity, you may have suffered more than your fair share of insensitivities and insults. You can learn to keep insults at bay and from hurting your inner self. Remind yourself that negative or hurtful comments do not define you, but your ability to rise above them does.

Action for the day:

Think of a recent time when someone made an offensive or insulting comment to you. In your journal, write about how the comment says more about the person who delivered it than about you.

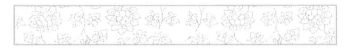

Break some eggs.

To make an omelet, you have to break some eggs, as the old saying goes. Think about the first human to have ever made an omelet. He probably made a lot of mistakes initially— throwing the whole egg onto the hot griddle, not mixing the eggs first, not flipping them over.

The only way we ever learn something new is when we give ourselves the freedom to screw up. There are probably a number of new things you've always longed to try, but you felt your weight got in the way. So do them now. Sign up for fiddle lessons. Give square dancing a try. Learn to crochet. Sure, your family will ask you to practice fiddle in a sound-proof room for a while, and you'll be stepping on toes and colliding with bodies during those first few barn dances. But WLS has given you a new lease on life, and now is the time to expand your horizons. It's never too late to learn.

Action for the day:

Pick one activity you have always wanted to try. Pull out the yellow pages and find a local community center or school that offers lessons and call them.

Yield.

There's a saying that ought to be taught to all driver's education students—the right of way cannot be taken, it can only
be given. It really doesn't matter if you had the right of way
at that intersection. If the other driver has no intention of
yielding, the only thing you'll accomplish by pulling ahead is
a dented fender at best and a totaled car and injuries at worst.

That's good advice in other areas of life as well. Some people
are not well-meaning, and will do everything in their power
to draw you into a fight. They may have disagreed with your
choice to get WLS. They may want to undermine your efforts
to maintain a healthy WLS lifestyle. Whatever their motives,
learn to recognize them. And once you do, learn to walk away
from any ensuing arguments. They don't want to negotiate;
they just want to fight. Taking them up on that will only lead
to bruised feelings.

Action for the day:

Think about the people you encounter on a regular basis who
are always trying to draw you into arguments. Begin to develop strategies for avoiding these conflicts, whether by changing the subject or even walking away.

Enjoy your food.

Sometimes it feels like food is the enemy. But you can't give up eating altogether. You still can be passionate about food and flavors. Your passion for food just needs to be redirected a little to make dishes that are small, healthy, and, just as importantly, tasty. Don't settle for unsatisfying or bland.

Have you noticed the first bite always tastes the best? You are not missing out on the best part of the meal by eating less. Rather than having seconds, develop the habit of having a particularly good meal again soon, or even for breakfast and lunch the next day. Learning to adjust your passion for food to your new lifestyle is crucial for maintaining long-term weight loss.

Action for the day:

Make a favorite meal today. Be sure to especially savor the first couple of bites. Stop eating at your first sign of fullness, knowing you can have another serving at your next mealtime.

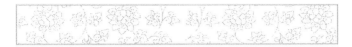

Don't get too hungry.

Getting too hungry can be a form of self-sabotage. When you allow yourself to get really hungry, it is much harder to make good food choices. It is harder to care about what you are putting in your mouth. It is much easier to choose something that is instantly gratifying and unhealthy.

So, eat enough and eat frequently enough that you don't get too hungry. Remember that eating less is not necessarily equated with losing weight. Eating enough is a better approach. Then, your metabolism will stay revved up and you won't get too hungry. Space your meals a bit closer together, and add protein-based snacks in your day if you know it will be a long time before your next meal.

Action for the day:

Make a food plan today that will keep you from getting too hungry. See how you do. Tomorrow, make a food plan based on what you learned today.

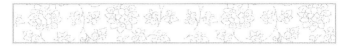

Be realistic.

While many WLS patients wish they could be at some magical weight they consider ideal, the weight you choose needs to be realistic. Not necessarily what you weighed in college or when you got married. Not necessarily less than your sister.

Are you shooting for a weight that you can live with, even if it doesn't match the "magic number" you long to see on the scale? Are you capable of performing your desired activities? Are you healthy? Can you maintain the necessary lifestyle in order to maintain your ideal weight?

Action for the day:

Think about your definition of an ideal weight. Are you aiming for a realistic number you can maintain? If not, explore why not. You could be sabotaging your success.

Be kind to your body.

When you hit a plateau, it's easy to become frustrated. You want your body to keep losing. You may contemplate extreme measures. But you need to let your body "catch its breath," so to speak. Think of it like pouring water from a pitcher into a funnel. You eventually want to empty the whole pitcher, but every once in awhile you need to pause and let the funnel drain. That plateau gives your organs and your skin and your soul a chance to adjust to the change.

And give yourself a chance, too. Do you recognize that face in the mirror? More than just your body is changing. Your mind is absorbing the change, too. Breathe deeply. Take time out to celebrate your progress, and know it will continue in your body's own time.

Action for the day:

Think of plateaus as time your body and mind need to adjust to the big changes you are going through. For today, be kind with your body and love it through its changes.

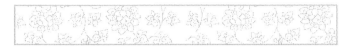

Avoid the L.G.M.

Everyone has met "perfect" people before. There are some
people who—at least outwardly—appear able to accomplish
great things at work, maintain impeccable health and raise a
ridiculously happy family. And some of them aren't faking or
hiding horrible secrets—they really are blessed in many ways.
No matter how tempting it is, do not allow yourself to wallow
in jealousy. It can lead to nothing positive.

If the "picture perfect" person is a friend of yours, it's even
more important to avoid the L.G.M. (Little Green Monster).
Jealousy has a tendency to push people away. And pushing
away a successful friend can deprive you of much-needed
support—not to mention a cheering section for when you
accomplish a goal. Successful people didn't get that way on
their own. They had the support and goodwill of friends
along the way.

Action for the day:

Instead of comparing yourself to someone else today, look at
how far you have come on your WLS journey and encourage
yourself.

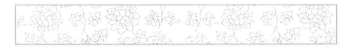

Treat your emotions as clues.

The best solution for emotional eating is for you to become
an ace detective. Treat your emotions as intriguing mysteries
to be solved, not pains to be numbed. Your long-term weight
loss depends on it.

By calling your emotions "clues" instead of "crises" you can
discover your emotional-eating triggers and develop an
action strategy (like journaling or calling a friend) instead of
a reaction response (yelling at your family or indulging in an
unhealthy food to get rid of your strong emotion).

Action for the day:

For today, treat your emotions as clues. Instead of reacting
to your emotions, take a look at them individually and ask
yourself, "What is this emotion trying to tell me?"

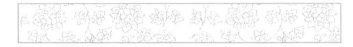

Ask for directions.

You may think all necessary WLS information was given to you during that initial phase when you began your WLS process. You may feel as though there isn't anything else you can learn at this point. But remember: medical research leads to new findings all the time, and if you are not consistently asking questions, you may as well be driving around in circles.

It can be humbling to ask for "directions"—it makes you feel inadequate and you may worry that others think you are weak or incapable of figuring things out for yourself. Swallow your pride and seek advice from trusted experts. You may find that new roads were constructed while you were looking elsewhere.

Action for the day:

Identify one WLS-related issue that has been concerning you lately, and research up-to-date answers from trusted sources.

Don't bunt.

Before WLS, you probably tried every diet in the book—and then some. You undoubtedly withstood a phenomenal amount of abuse. Many people struggling with obesity spend a good part of their lives in shame. Even after you reach your goal weight, it may be hard for you to appreciate your perseverance and victory in light of your past scars that you continue to carry with you. Don't let those scars slow you down. Now is not the time to hold back.

You were not put here on this earth to make a sacrifice bunt for other players. You were put here to accomplish extraordinary things. Step up to the plate! Even if you occasionally hit a fly ball, or only manage a single, one of your hits is bound to be a homer. Every single attempt you make could be your next home run, so act accordingly.

Action for the day:

Whatever is on your task list for today, make a vow to do each thing with gusto. Whether it's washing the car or finishing up that project at work, knock it out of the park!

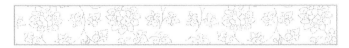

Compare yourself to…yourself.

How many times have you been intimidated by someone who holds a higher societal position than you? Whether it's a "higher-up" at work or anyone else who has a "bigger" job or higher salary, we all feel puny in comparison to someone else at least once in life. But why do you feel that someone with a more impressive job title or fancier car is better than you? At the end of the day, that person goes home to a family life just as complicated as yours, maybe even more so. He may be surrounded by leather seats and a stereo system, but he still gets stuck in the same traffic jams as you. And he may very well feel intimidated by people who occupy a station above his.

Allowing yourself to be intimidated only thwarts your efforts at reaching your dreams. Try not to compare your life to another's. We are all in the same boat; we all suffer misfortunes, and we all struggle with day-to-day life.

Action for the day:

Write in your journal one accomplishment for which you are truly proud. Reflect on that accomplishment, knowing that you are strong enough to do even more.

Make "right decisions" a goal.

Do you set goals and track your progress? It's a well-known
fact that you are more likely to reach a goal if you write it
down and monitor your growth.

If you've been struggling to make good choices, make "making
good choices" your goal. Create a chart, and put a star or
other positive symbol on the days you make good and
healthy choices. By tracking your right decisions, you'll see
them increase.

Action for the day:

Make a "right decisions" chart. In your journal, start a list of
the right decisions you make. Looking back on the challenges
you have overcome will inspire you.

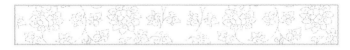

Pet your pet.

Sometimes all you really need is an understanding soul to spend time with you while you're dealing with difficult issues. Friends and family can obviously fulfill that need. But if you don't really feel like talking, and you just need to sit quietly in the company of another, don't underestimate the power of a pet to play that role for you.

Research has shown that pet owners are mentally and physically healthier than those who do not own pets. Everyone who has ever owned a dog knows the joy of coming home from a hard day and being greeted by a family member who is genuinely thrilled to see you and makes no demands on you—other than a pat on the head, a belly rub, or the chance to curl up at your feet. And as an added bonus, dogs serve as great motivators to get out and walk.

Action for the day:

If you don't own a pet, do some research today on what kind of pet would fit into your lifestyle best. If you already own a pet, when you get home tonight, put aside all your work and simply bask in the unconditional love that only animals can give.

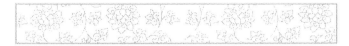

Declutter your life.

Everything has its place: books belong on bookshelves, not stacked up on your bedside table; plates and food belong in the kitchen, not on the coffee table; your work papers belong in your office, not strewn all over the living room.

Clutter can be a huge distraction and can undermine your serenity and your goals. It can inhibit your care after WLS. Instead, maintaining a sense of order in the house will help you maintain a sense of order in your life.

Action for the day:

Today, go through your house and find 20 items to donate to charity. Ask a friend to help if you think this will be too hard to do alone.

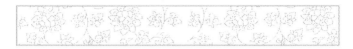

Win an Oscar.

People like to talk about the "overnight stars" who suddenly become the most recognized faces in Hollywood. These people supposedly step off the bus and within hours have agents and major movie roles. But it rarely happens that way. The actors we suddenly notice have likely been kicking around for years, taking bit parts, working in dinner theatre, and waiting tables. As with any lofty goal, the behind-the-scenes work is backbreaking and exhausting, and most people don't notice the efforts you're putting in.

Diligence now will reap great rewards in the long run—you'll arrive at your goal stronger and more capable. Don't despair if it's not happening overnight. The rare overnight sensations tend to burn out quickly—your goal isn't 15 minutes of fame, but the Oscar.

Action for the day:

Write in your journal about one long-term goal you would like to achieve. Reflect on the hard work that will be involved, and accept the fact that there will be no short cut.

September

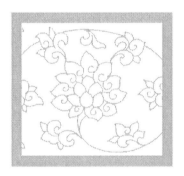

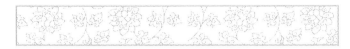

Write your hurts in the sand—but your blessings in stone.

The way you handle the hurts you have been dealt speaks to your ability to forgive and move on. When you dwell on past hurts, you can stay in a victim mindset and look for more hurt. Constantly expecting the negative can cause you to hold back from situations that may in fact turn out wonderfully. Looking for hurt can make you blind to the good things in your life.

At those times when people say or do things that hurt you, try to write those memories in the sand—allow the passage of time to blow them away. Your blessings, on the other hand, should be carved in stone so that you can appreciate them during the times when you are feeling overwhelmed.

Action for the day:

Make a list of all of the special things and people in your life that provide you with a firm anchor—your family, friends, faith, health, career. Whatever gives you strength, celebrate it.

Take the plunge—now.

There are people who put off getting married because they need more time to prepare or who agonize over whether to start a family because they are not quite ready. Some won't change jobs because they feel their skills are lacking.

Of course, once people take the plunge—whether by marrying, having a baby, or switching jobs—they discover that they were right! They weren't completely prepared. But with that knowledge comes the revelation that nobody is ever really ready. Relationships, families, careers all require constant effort, and you are always learning something new— both about yourself and others. Putting things off because you are waiting for the right time is self-defeating. Resign yourself to the fact that conditions will never be absolutely perfect. Just muster your courage and take that first step.

Action for the day:

Today, take a step in the direction you feel drawn toward, even if you don't feel completely ready.

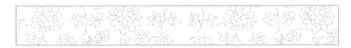

Practice relaxation techniques.

Living a healthy, happy WLS lifestyle takes effort—daily
effort. But it doesn't have to be a constant uphill battle.
Even if you occasionally slip, you won't be starting at the
beginning. Viewing your life as a constant struggle will only
accomplish one thing—you will convince yourself that
only Superman could stay on track, and then, that lack of
confidence will make your job much harder.

You are succeeding. You will continue to succeed by using
your tools. One great tool is relaxation. Rather than obsessing
over a task and making it seem bigger than it is, relax
and lower your stress level. It will make your journey more
pleasant without compromising your goals.

Action for the day:

Try some relaxation techniques. You don't have to know how
to meditate. Simply take five minutes to sit, close your eyes,
breathe deeply, and try to clear your mind. Practice daily
until it becomes second nature.

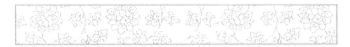

Read the writing on the wall.

Perhaps you're afraid of setting new boundaries with a friend or family member, who doesn't quite understand your WLS needs, for fear of angering them. So, you're avoiding the confrontation and hoping the problem goes away by itself. Meanwhile, you're inadvertently dismissing warning signs that things may well be coming to a head regardless.

Pay close attention to the clues around you if you want to head problems off at the pass. Pretending nothing is wrong won't alleviate your conflict. It will simply prevent you from reading the road signs ahead and may lead you to a crash.

Action for the day:

If you have been putting off a discussion with a friend or family member for fear of angering them, make plans to have that discussion the next time you are together. Rehearse your discussion with a safe friend, if necessary.

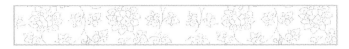

Take your time; Rome wasn't built in a day.

So, have you reached your goal weight yet? Are you well into your successful maintenance period? Of course, you've resolved all of your emotional issues and are now a phenomenally healthy model of happy, successful living, right? Well, don't despair; as they say, Rome wasn't built in a day. Nothing worth accomplishing can be achieved overnight. If it could, it wouldn't be much of an accomplishment, right?

Patience is a difficult virtue to cultivate, especially in this fast-paced society that extols overnight success. Even a year or more after your surgery, you may not be exactly where you want to be. But that's okay. Your life is not meant to be rushed. It's a slowly-unfolding story. Savor it and know that you are doing your best to make sure that the next chapter holds even more promise.

Action for the day:

Reflect on all that you have accomplished so far, both the momentous and the "small." Meditate on what your next chapter will hold.

Wherever you go, be there.

Buddhists practice a technique called "mindfulness," the idea that your attention should be focused on the present rather than on what is to come. Focusing can be easy enough to do if the current task is all-consuming. But what about when you are washing the dishes? Or ironing? Or eating? Sometimes, it's easy to let your mind wander.

True mindfulness demands that your full attention be placed on the activity at hand. That means that the only thing going through your mind at the dinner table is how nice the food smells and how the third bite doesn't taste as good as the first. Practicing mindfulness helps keep obsessive food thoughts at bay when you are not supposed to be eating, and creates more satisfaction when you are.

Action for the day:

At meal times today, focus only on eating your meal. Focus on the colors, textures, and smells. If other thoughts try to barge in, refocus immediately on the activity at hand.

Use your bed wisely.

Of course, you know that a consistent good night's sleep
gives you the energy you need to face the day refreshed and
energetic. Turning your bedroom into a multi-purpose room
can have a profound negative effect. Most sleep experts
recommend that people refrain from watching television,
reading, or eating while in bed. There are only two things for
which a bed should be used, and if you go beyond that, one
of those things—sleep—will suffer.

Whether you're watching TV, reading, or checking your
Blackberry while in bed, there is something about lounging in
it that is conducive to snacking. And because your mind is
focused on the television or the printed word, you may find
yourself snacking without really thinking about it. Make your
bedroom a sanctuary away from food.

Action for the day:

If there is a television in your bedroom, consider moving it
out. And today, eat your meals in the kitchen or dining room.

Be humbled by your gift.

If you have reached your goal weight and are well into the
maintenance period, you may be tempted to revert to some
old habits. After all, you met your goal; why not celebrate a
little? Be careful. Indulging in old thinking patterns can have
devastating consequences.

Always be aware that WLS demands a life-long effort that you
can never abandon. Remember that you have been given a
great gift through WLS, but that gift requires your constant
attention. You have not been magically "fixed." The next time
you start to entertain some of these old thinking patterns,
cling to the gift that you have been given.

Action for the day:

Write in your journal about what you feel are the greatest
gifts you've received because of WLS, and reflect on ways to
keep enjoying those gifts.

Schedule fewer activities.

Do you find yourself practically living in your car—picking the oldest up at school and dropping him off at basketball practice, running back to school to pick up your middle child's homework, picking up the dry cleaning and the groceries, running the dog to the vet, and finishing with just enough time to do it all again tomorrow?

There's nothing wrong with scheduling a few activities that your kids enjoy. But there's something terribly wrong with having so many different activities that everyone burns out—especially you. So, if carving out time to take care of yourself means telling each child to pick just one outside activity, then so be it. They have a lifetime to try new activities. But they have only one shot at seeing the role model of a healthy, fulfilled parent.

Action for the day:

Spend time today making a list of all of your family's activities and obligations. Then, sit down with them this evening and work on culling down that list. As hard as it is, you will all benefit from this activity.

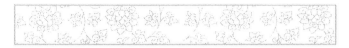

Focus on the joy.

In almost any given moment, you have a choice. You can pick out "what's wrong with that picture," or you can look for what's right. As you walk into your kitchen, your first thought can be, "I hate it when my husband doesn't wipe up his crumbs," or you can think, "I love how sunny this room is."

Negative thinking can become a well-worn habit, but it never brings peace of mind. Looking for what you like will bring you much more joy.

Action for the day:

Police your thoughts today. Whenever you lead with a negative thought, back up and start again with something positive—something joyous.

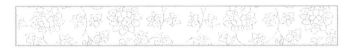

Develop tranquility.

Stress, as you know all too well, can easily lead to weight gain and the overall sabotage of your WLS lifestyle. Yet, many WLS patients simply don't know how to deal with this potentially harmful emotion.

There are many effective and natural means of reducing stress that don't cost a penny, including nature walks, deep breathing, enhancing sleep quality, relaxation exercises, meditation, visualization, and guided imagery.

Action for the day:

Choose an activity that will reduce your stress, and engage in it today.

Use small tools.

Have you noticed that serving spoons have been getting bigger? It's true—some silverware companies are now increasing
the size of the utensils they manufacture. Talk about sabotage!

Taking small bites is one great tool for maintaining control of
how much you eat. Did you know that you can now find
small spoons (in the baby aisle) to take with you wherever
you go? Small bites, chewed slowly and thoroughly, will keep
overeating in check—whether you use the little disposable
spoons, cocktail forks, or other small utensils.

Action for the day:

Have you lapsed into taking larger bites and eating faster?
For today, use small utensils, and chew slowly and thoroughly.
You'll probably be more satisfied than you expect.

September *13*

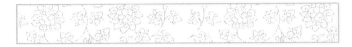

Be realistic.

Are you a perfectionist? Do you tend to give up and overeat if you can't be perfect with your food? The reality is making one mistake does not mean you have to throw in the towel.

You don't have to be perfect; just be honest with yourself. When you start to tell yourself you're a hopeless case, stop and ask yourself: "Is that really true? Am I really hopeless?"

Action for the day:

Be realistic and admit there are things you can do to help yourself and your situation. Today, make a new choice and get moving in a healthier direction.

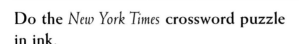

Do the *New York Times* crossword puzzle in ink.

Doing a difficult crossword puzzle in pencil may seem like a smart approach. If you make a mistake, you can simply erase the answer and try again. But having that option paves the way to making impulsive choices. And after awhile, too many erasures will make the puzzle illegible. When you write the answers in pen, you're committing yourself.

Now take that approach to your life as a whole. Try to avoid rash decisions you'll regret later. Take your time. Do research. Develop a plan. Know the likely consequences. Then, write it in ink.

Action for the day:

In your journal, write about a recent rash decision you made that did not turn out as well as you would have liked. Then, imagine how the situation would have unfolded if you had taken the time to think things through and develop a plan of action you could feel confident about. Resolve to act more deliberately next time.

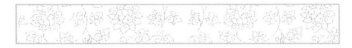

Harbor hope.

So what do you do when you stumble? Do you shake your head in self-disgust and say to yourself, "Well, what else is new? I always screw up. What's the point?" Or...do you humbly acknowledge the fact that you are a flawed human being (like everyone else on the planet) and vow to do better next time?

If you "slam" yourself too much, you'll lose hope for the future. Hope is your heart's way of pushing you to try more, accomplish more, and be more. Don't extinguish that spark.

Action for the day:

Reflect on the most recent misstep you made in your WLS lifestyle. Determine what lesson can be learned from it, forgive yourself for it, and then move on.

Know thyself.

Knowing what you are capable of and what you are likely to struggle with will help tremendously in your efforts to stay on the path to WLS success. If there are situations that are challenging to you, acknowledge that. You have nothing to prove to anyone by ignoring your limitations and pushing forward. And having difficulties in certain areas does not make you weak.

If you know that office parties are your downfall, you need to accept that fact and then take the necessary steps to avoid them. If that means staying in your office or going home a little early, then so be it. Know your strengths and weaknesses and make your decisions based on them.

Action for the day:

Reflect on the situation you were in when you last stumbled—eating something you should not have, skipping your vitamins or water, etc. What can you learn about yourself from that situation? Apply that knowledge about yourself as you move forward.

White-knuckle it if you have to.

Making healthy choices just isn't going to be easy all the time. Some days you will find yourself eating the broccoli; other days you will be craving the chocolate. On the days when food thoughts are pushing you in the wrong direction, consider white-knuckling it through the craving.

When you white-knuckle your way through something, it's uncomfortable. But, you can handle some discomfort, right? And while white-knuckling it is not the preferred method for long-term recovery, it is a vital tool to pull you through when you need it.

Action for the day:

If you find yourself drawn to an unhealthy food or to overeating, pull out the tool of white-knuckling. It can get you through.

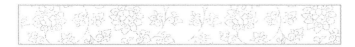

Cultivate willingness.

Two words, when added to your vocabulary, will change
your life: I WILL. When you say, "I will," you are making a
statement of action as well as commitment.

With all the temptations to eat or obsess about your food or
your body, an "I WILL" attitude can give you a clear advantage. If you take a misstep, and someone suggests a tool to try,
say, "I will." Don't say, "That won't work for me, because…"
or "I already tried that and…" or "I hate having to…." Simply
say, "I will." And then, do it.

Action for the day:

For today, add these two simple words to your vocabulary:
I WILL.

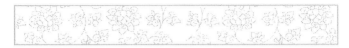

Let yourself be imperfect.

So, you don't understand the task your boss has asked you to do. You car needs a good cleaning and you have to drive a coworker to lunch. Your bills are due and you can't find your checkbook.

Being imperfect is stressful. But it's also human. Can you let yourself off the hook? Can you remind yourself that in the long run, you won't be remembered for the condition of your car? When you allow yourself to be human, you can let go of all kinds of stress—stress that might otherwise be a huge trigger for overeating.

Action for the day:

Give yourself a break from the self criticism today. If negative self talk creeps in, refocus your mind immediately on something positive. Allow yourself to be imperfect.

Resist the urge to feel good now.

Rather than feeling sad on Mother's Day, because you suffered the loss of a child, you buy a half gallon of ice cream and eat as much as you can—even if you get the dumping syndrome that comes with gastric bypass. Or…rather than feeling angry at your boss for denying your leave request for your family reunion, you crunch on potato chips—even if you feel ill afterwards.

No one likes to feel anxious, angry, or sad. But consider learning to sit with unpleasant emotions rather than eating over them. Literally stop, find a private place for a few minutes, sit and really allow yourself to feel the feeling, and know that it will pass—sooner than you think.

Action for the day:

In your journal, make a list of things you can do to help yourself feel your feelings. For example, you could put on your list, "Hug a pillow and cry my eyes out," or "Write down what I am feeling and thinking in my journal."

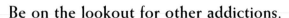

Be on the lookout for other addictions.

Many people who have WLS are addicted to food, especially sugar and refined carbs. When food is calling to you to the point of obsession, you are feeling the pull of an addiction. No matter how clearly you understand that eating in that moment is neither healthy nor physically necessary, you can't seem to stop yourself from doing it.

Sometimes after WLS, food addiction subsides. You stop eating foods that are most likely to cause an addictive response, and you see results that are inspiring. As the newness wears off, you try to avoid returning to compulsive eating, but in that moment you are vulnerable to other addictions. Other addictions can include alcohol, drugs, shopping, sex, gambling, and more. An addiction can control your life even when you are slimmer. So be on your guard, and get help immediately if you suspect you are becoming addicted to anything else (or turning back to food).

Action for the day:

Take a few minutes to consider the role of addiction in your life. Is there something that "owns" you? Something you need to consider letting go of?

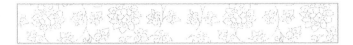

Forgive yourself.

You've had a tough road. Being obese was miserable. And you probably felt you were to blame, and that you should have been able to lose the weight and keep it off on your own. Maybe you understand the truth now: Obesity is a disease with many contributing factors. It is not a sign of a weak will. It is by far one of the most challenging and devastating diseases with which to deal.

Forgive yourself for your imperfections, and encourage yourself as you embrace your new lifestyle. WLS is not a cure for obesity, but it is a great opportunity. You'll be able to take much better advantage of it if you are not beating yourself up all the time.

Action for the day:

In your journal, write a letter of forgiveness to yourself. Tell yourself you understand how hard it's been, and that you are ready to finally forgive and move on.

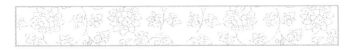

Give people the opportunity to understand.

Perhaps you grow tired at times of explaining to others what
you must do to maintain a healthy WLS lifestyle. You fear
that people will challenge or judge you on the choice you
made to have WLS. Undoubtedly, there are people who will
do that and sabotage your efforts to boot. However, know
that there are probably even more people who would be
understanding and supportive if they only knew what you
face each day.

There's no need to provide in-depth information to strangers
or mere acquaintances. But a little honesty with others in your
life could make your daily choices easier. If you simply cannot
attend that neighborhood holiday party because you do not
want to deal with the temptations, explain that. Give people
the opportunity to understand.

Action for the day:

If you have been putting off explaining to someone what you
need to do to remain healthy, do so today.

Play your part.

Everybody has a role to play in life. For some people, their destiny is to cure a disease or solve perplexing crimes. For others, destiny holds something a little simpler. Maybe your destiny is to touch and improve just one life by living a good example of a successful WLS lifestyle.

All destinies are important. Remember that any time you find yourself faced with a seemingly mundane task. Jobs that seem small while you're doing them can prove to be much bigger and more important than you think.

Action for the day:

Think of one mundane task that you have been putting off. Get it done today, and say a prayer of thanks that you are alive and well enough to do it.

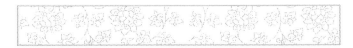

Be daring.

You have come far since your WLS. You have done what a few years ago seemed impossible—you took charge of your health and gave yourself a new lease on life.

Now is not the time to become timid. There is so much more you can—and will—accomplish. Overcoming obesity is just the beginning. Continue to harness the daring spirit that made all of this possible and embark on a new phase in your life. Nothing can stand in your way if you choose to dare.

Action for the day:

List the steps needed for the next "big" goal you have and begin taking the first steps today.

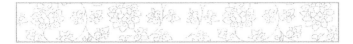

Act on your "impossible" dream.

Hopefully, by now you have made a list of goals that you can refer to every once in awhile. This will give you a nudge toward fulfilling them. Are most of the goals relatively minor?

It's fine to have those on the list, but try being a little bolder. Find a major goal—switching to a new career, finishing up a degree, buying a new house, starting your own business, traveling around the world. Don't put off putting it on your goals list just because it is daunting. That's the reason it SHOULD be on your list. It will give you the courage to tackle it, and as you check off the "smaller" goals, you will see how achievable "the big one" really is.

Action for the day:

Think of the biggest, most audacious goal you have and write it down.

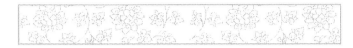

Expect royal treatment.

Being famous, being born into the right family, being thin, or being rich doesn't make someone a better human being, or more worthy of respect. You deserve the same kind of respect as the Queen of England.

Don't be afraid to demand respect. When you allow someone to treat you as unimportant or unworthy of their attention, time, or effort, you are not being fair to yourself, nor are you being honest about your true worth.

Action for the day:

Do not allow yourself to be treated with disrespect—even if that means calling someone on their disrespectful behavior.

Do what works.

It's easy to get caught up in the drama of being out of control with eating. That familiar feeling of giving in pushes your dreams of getting healthy and slimmer further out of sight.

Resist giving in. There are strategies that can work for you if you choose to use them. So, instead of repeating an old pattern of behavior that does not work, try another strategy that might. Keep trying different strategies until you find what works.

Action for the day:

Today, try using a proven strategy to help you stay on track— one you've used before or a new one. Put aside your resistance and see what happens.

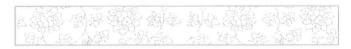

Live today.

Some people are too impatient for the finish line. They develop such tunnel vision that they fail to enjoy—or learn lessons from—the journey itself. Living life in "the now" seems a waste of time.

But the destination is only part of your life. You will reach it eventually. In the meantime, try to enjoy the ride. Who knows? You may even discover some back roads that take you to new, unimaginable destinations.

Action for the day:

Throughout the day, ask yourself one question: "What's joyful in my life—right now? "

Minimize damage.

Because you aren't perfect, there may be a time when you want to eat more than you need. Before you take an extra bite, try to distract yourself. Get busy and put off eating.

But, when you do eat—especially if you are overeating—pick foods that will satisfy you without adding a lot of calories. (For example, try celery sticks versus crackers, chicken or shrimp versus pepperoni.)

Action for the day:

Write down a plan of action for the days when you are tempted to overeat. By developing a list of healthy foods that satisfy you, you can minimize the damage of eating more than you need. And if you are consistently overeating, seek help from a professional.

October

Take care of the big stuff first.

A professor asked his students to guess how many rocks could fit into a glass jar he held. To find out, he placed many small pebbles into the jar. But then, he realized, the bigger rocks didn't fit in. Next, he did the reverse—he placed the biggest rocks in first and then added the pebbles. A surprising number of pebbles fit into the crevices between the larger rocks.

The bigger rocks symbolize the really important things in your life—your health, your family, and your faith. Focus on making sure those big rocks are in place before you start to add the pebbles. When you fill your jar with pebbles, the big rocks won't fit.

Action for the day:

Write down a short list of the truly important things in your life. Then write a second list of things that you may enjoy or want to do, but that you could drop occasionally without major suffering. Put the second list away and vow not to look at it until you've addressed the first list.

Purr while you nap.

A cat knows how to lounge in a sunbeam without guilt or
how to ask for attention without shame. A cat will lie in your
lap, sleeping and purring at the same time. They understand
what pleases them and they seek it out. Not only that, they
know they are entitled to it, and they revel in it.

Do you know how to purr while you nap? How to feel so
satisfied, relaxed, comfortable, pleased, and nurtured you can't
help but feel bliss? Do you deny yourself those feelings?

Action for the day:

Today, be a cat. Spend a few minutes seeking true bliss. Take
a luxurious nap, get a massage, lounge in a warm bath, or
read a book while curled up on the couch.

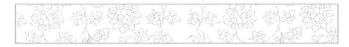

Think about the bottom line.

Days can be so busy for some people they never stop to
think about what they are doing and how it is affecting them.
But to make changes in your lifestyle, thinking is critical.
Most important is thinking about your bottom line—your
deepest goals.

Each day, you can look back and think about what you did
and how it will impact your bottom-line goals. Thus,
developing the habit of making a connection between what
you say you want and what you actually do.

Action for the day:

Spend some quiet time thinking about your day. How much
of what you did contributed to you reaching your bottom-line
goals? How much of what you did will detract from your
goals?

Stay in touch with your surgeon.

Many WLS patients lose touch with their surgeons over time.
Several reasons account for this. Once some patients figure
out their program, they think they are all set. They're on top
of the world. So, they rationalize they won't need to stay in
contact with their surgeon. Others are struggling, but are
simply too embarrassed to ask for help.

Either way, staying in touch with your surgeon is a good idea.
If new research shows you need a certain lab test or a new
supplement, your surgeon can advise you. In addition, your
surgeon just might be able to help you with a WLS-related
problem. (What if your surgery is "broken," for example? Or,
you are vitamin deficient?) Finally, the more records exist
regarding WLS patients, the more accurate research regarding
outcomes and treatment options will be.

Action for the day:

If you're due for a check-up or if you are having problems,
schedule an appointment with your surgeon today.

Talk to yourself.

When you are struck with the urge to eat when you're not hungry, you are wanting to eat for emotional reasons. Before you act on an urge to eat for reasons other than hunger, first have a little conversation with yourself.

Ask yourself, "What am I feeling right now?" "What do I really want?" "Is there anything I need right now?" Then listen. Really listen to yourself and respond with kindness to your real need.

Action for the day:

Today, if you get hit with the urge to eat when you're not hungry, in your journal ask yourself the above questions and answer them. Then, take positive action.

Go the way of the snail.

When you are faced with exciting food that you worry you won't be able to stop eating, use the "Snail Strategy." Eat slowly. S-L-O-W-L-Y.

Take small bites and chew thoroughly, then pause for a bit before the next bite. If you slow down your eating, you will get satisfied on less food. When everyone else is finished, you will have eaten much less than you would have otherwise. You never know when a strategy will work for you, so give it a try.

Action for the day:

Slow down today. Just for this day chew slowly and allow more time between bites. See how that affects your satisfaction.

Take some risks with your wardrobe.

Are you still buying baggy clothes that hide your shape? Or, solid colors to mask your weight? Adjusting to a new body size takes time. It can take two years or more before you can see the actual body you have in your mind's eye.

When you're out getting new clothes, try on some things you never would have considered before. You may surprise yourself.

Action for the day:

Make a date to go shopping with a friend or relative who will give you moral support while you try on some new clothes. Try on styles you would never have considered in the past and see how you feel.

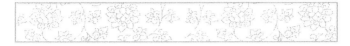

Put an end to the rebellion.

After years of dieting and deprivation, many WLS patients struggle with feelings of rebellion when they are told to follow the new WLS lifestyle.

You might resist making a food plan or recording what you eat. You might not want to measure foods that are easy to overeat. Perhaps you skip exercise because you were forced to exercise as a child. While rebellious feelings are normal, they are ultimately self destructive. Rethink your rebellion. Is it worth it?

Action for the day:

Take a firm stance with yourself. When your rebellious nature tries to take control, refuse to allow it.

Eschew perfection.

It's not uncommon for people who have food addiction to try to eat perfectly, fail, and then give up. If you're in that vicious cycle, you know how disappointing it is to try hard, slip up a little, and then throw in the towel. You've probably done it so many times you almost don't feel like trying again anymore.

As hard as it sounds, you can begin to deal with this problem by actively resisting perfection. Do everything imperfectly. Always leave a bite on your plate. Part your hair crooked on purpose. Spell something wrong. Be late. Don't send a greeting card. Make everyone go to the movie you want to see. Let your linens sit in the dryer and put them on the beds wrinkled. Leave crumbs on the table. Avoid perfection as a rule, and learn how to live in the gray areas of life.

Action for the day:

Do three things imperfectly today, on purpose. Write about how it feels in your journal.

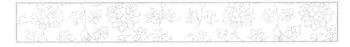

Schedule nothing.

After WLS, a person's energy level often goes up quite a bit. It's a joy to have the energy and ability to do all the things you've wanted to do for years, but were unable to. Just because you can now, though, doesn't mean you have to. When you get going too fast, important self-care habits get skipped, and your WLS recovery suffers.

So, schedule some time to do nothing. Stay in your jammies all day and watch TV. Or, go to the library for the afternoon and read. Or, sleep in really late. Whatever your definition of "nothing" is, make time for it in your life.

Action for the day:

Look at your calendar and block out time for a "nothing" morning, afternoon, or entire day as soon as you can.

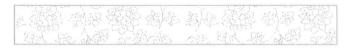

Eat enough.

Many people who struggle with weight have a history of dieting, restricting, cutting back. You probably feel like you're doing a good thing when you eat less. And when you up your intake, you feel guilty.

Sometimes, though, people who have WLS develop a "food is bad" attitude that undermines their weight loss. If you don't eat enough calories, your body will think you are starving it and hold on to the weight. The lack of calories causes your metabolism to slow and your weight loss to stall.

Action for the day:

Review the guidelines your surgeon and/or nutritionist have given you. (If you don't have recommended dietary guidelines, get them.) Find out how much you need to be eating to achieve your weight goal. Also, write down what you eat today and calculate the calories. Are you eating enough?

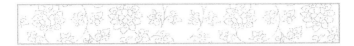

Be uncomfortable.

Just for today, don't do one thing you really want to do—or—
do one thing you really don't want to do. Practice being
uncomfortable. Sit with feelings that you otherwise might
try to avoid by eating.

Many of the problems weight loss surgery patients run into
stem from the inability to say "NO!" to themselves—their
unwillingness to sit with uncomfortable feelings.

Action for the day:

Allow yourself to be uncomfortable today by saying "no" to
yourself. Then, record your experience and feelings in your
journal.

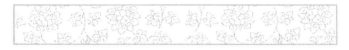

Admit what you know.

Sometimes you know you are struggling with food, but can't quite figure out why. Often, the answer is right in front of you.

If you are feeling out of control, take a "bird's eye view." Imagine you are flying way up high, viewing your problem from afar. Can you see better what is getting in the way of your success?

Action for the day:

If you are having a bad food day—but don't really know why—take a few minutes to sit quietly, breathe, and imagine looking at your problem from a distance. If you already know what the problem is and how to remedy it, admit it to yourself today and make a plan of action.

Be like Pollyanna.

We can learn a lot from characters in children's stories. Take Pollyanna, for example. If you haven't heard the story, it's about a young girl who endures many hardships, yet she still finds something to be happy about. She calls it, "The Glad Game."

Have you tried playing The Glad Game? Sometimes negative thinking is simply a habit. People often act more like Eeyore than Pollyanna. But, you don't have to.

Action for the day:

Whether you feel like it or not, play The Glad Game today. When you feel like complaining, find something to be glad about instead.

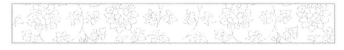

Change your course—even if just by one degree.

When a pilot is off course, he or she can make a tiny correction and set the plane on a new course. You can do that with your life. If you are headed somewhere you don't want to go, change course.

The great thing is you only have to make a small change to impact your life significantly. A one-degree turn will take you to a totally different place.

Action for the day:

Make a small, permanent change today that helps you to move in a healthier direction.

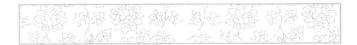

Stick with the winners.

As you look around your WLS support group, or think about your acquaintances and friends, you'll notice that some people are meeting their goals and some aren't. Some people are complaining and doing nothing about their problems. Some are working hard to live in the solution.

When someone lives in the solution it means they are actively acknowledging their challenge and practicing a new way to deal with it. They are finding solutions that might work, trying them, tweaking, and trying again. And they are moving forward. They are winning.

Action for the day:

Identify someone who is living in the solution to their problem. Give them a call today or initiate a conversation. Resolve to stick with the winners.

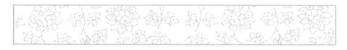

Have a "wacky-day plan."

Life is not always predictable. You wear a new fall sweater to work and the temperature climbs to 80 degrees. You plan a weekend away, and you get the flu. For WLS patients, unexpected events can ruin a good plan for the day. For example, you get delayed by a client, and by the time you finally get home you are so hungry you choose a quick, refined carbohydrate to eat.

When you get hit with a wacky day, have in place a "wacky day plan" so you don't get off track. For example, some people keep the fixings for a protein drink in their car for emergency situations.

Action for the day:

Make a "wacky-day plan." What will you do to protect your healthy way of life when something unpredictable happens?

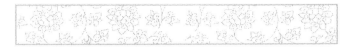

Burn the candle at one end.

With all that new-found energy, have you gotten too busy for your own good? Just because you can, doesn't mean you should. Burning the candle at both ends can lead to a quick burnout.

Be active and live your life, but give yourself time to relax and get centered, too. Find balance, and your candle will burn for a good, long time.

Action for the day:

Rather than overscheduling and overdoing, which can conflict with your desire to be healthy, give yourself some down time—some time to take care of you.

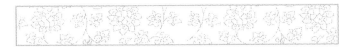

Use gratitude to get out of discouragement.

Have you ever felt so discouraged you sought comfort in overeating or other compulsive behaviors?

During your discouragement, try summoning up some gratitude. When you are eating compulsively and fearing you will regain your weight, self loathing or other negative emotions will not help. Nurture an attitude of gratitude so that even in hard times, even when you are getting sucked under in a raging swirl of discouragement, you are focusing on the way out.

Action for the day:

No matter how you feel today, write down five things for which you are grateful.

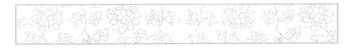

Get busy.

If you are a boredom eater, it's time to find something to do instead of eat.

Motivating yourself to do something different can be a challenge, but it is possible. What do you like to do? Maybe you like puzzles or clean closets. Do your bushes need pruning? Has it been a long time since you went to the library (where there is no food) to browse?

Action for the day:

Just for today, don't give in to boredom. Get busy.

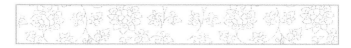

Believe you'll get better.

If you make an effort to do something every single day, no matter how awkward you are at the start, you'll get better at it. You have to. You couldn't walk when you first started out so long ago. Now you walk all the time. It's not a big deal.

It takes time and practice to establish new, healthier habits. But, have faith you will get better.

Action for the day:

Be conscious today of the new habits you are creating and practice them.

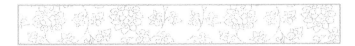

Stretch.

Are you happy with everything in your life? Is there
something you are dissatisfied with, but you haven't done
much about it? It's time to stretch. It's time to try a solution to
what's bugging you that is outside of your comfort zone.

People tend to want predictable lives—even if their lives are
dissatisfying to some degree. Learning new skills, the fear of
looking silly, not wanting to take the time, all these things
make change hard—but change anyway.

Action for the day:

Do something today that is a stretch for you. Something
that will move you closer to the satisfaction you are looking
for in life.

Consider your surroundings.

As your WLS lifestyle is not that of a hermit, consider the surroundings in which you live, work, and play.

Do you spend a lot of time in your kitchen at home or near food at work? Are you likely to suggest meeting a friend at a restaurant, rather than for a walk? Food is not evil, but if you love it a little too much, consider the surroundings in which you put yourself. Are you around food more than necessary?

Action for the day:

Pay attention to your surroundings today. Do you spend more time near food temptations than is healthy for you?

Listen to that little voice.

Life can be so busy and distracting, it's easy to ignore yourself. Sometimes ignoring yourself can become a habit. You just don't stop and pay attention to that little voice inside of you that is saying, "What I really need is...."

When you don't pay attention to yourself and your own needs, you are actively sabotaging your dream to lose weight and keep it off—whether you realize it or not.

Action for the day:

Sit quietly for a few minutes and ask yourself, "What do I need to be healthy and content?" Ask over and over again until you have at least one idea. Then, take action to move toward fulfilling that need.

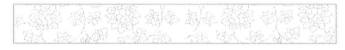

Let your adult self take charge.

Who are you going to bring with you as you move from
holiday event to holiday event in the coming months? Are
you going to bring the little child inside who hates being
deprived? Or, are you bringing with you the satisfied and
goal-oriented adult who will take care of your true needs?

When your inner child is in charge, you are more at risk for
making unhealthy choices. The inner child may be rebellious,
choosing to eat the things that are "forbidden." Your inner
adult is better at delaying gratification and thinking through
the consequences of a choice. When you are going into a
challenging situation, your adult self will be your best friend.
That part of you will say, "no," and will guide you onto an
exciting new path of success.

Action for the day:

Pay attention to the voices inside your head that help you
make choices as you go through your day. Identify your inner
child's influence, acknowledge it, and then gently allow your
inner adult to have the final say.

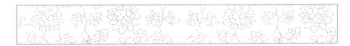

Get "religion."

Do you take your vitamins only when they occur to you? Are you unlikely to remember to bring your calcium with you for the day or to take your iron supplement in a way that will allow for the best absorption?

If you are going to be a zealot about anything, your vitamins and supplements are one of the best things you can choose. Unless you meet someone with a deficiency, or you develop one yourself, you may not realize how horrible one can be— or how permanent the damage.

Action for the day:

If you are not getting in all your vitamins and supplements, make a checklist to use—and use it. No excuses. Take your vitamins religiously.

Track your progress.

One of the most motivating things to use is a simple tracking sheet. Whether you want to lose weight, maintain a weight loss, take your vitamins, or exercise consistently, tracking your progress could be surprisingly motivating.

Post your tracking sheet somewhere where you'll see it often and experience the satisfaction of seeing progress build over time.

Action for the day:

Often people think something sounds like a good idea, but then they skip doing it. So instead of just thinking about it, today make a tracking sheet and start tracking an important goal.

Treat yourself.

You have chosen a new way of life with WLS—a new way
that isn't supposed to include a lot of unhealthy eating. But as
Halloween approaches, and other holidays follow close
behind, your senses will be assaulted more and more with
holiday treats. Are they really treats, though? When you look
at a piece of candy and think, "Oh, that looks good. One
won't hurt," you are not contemplating treating yourself, you
are contemplating sabotaging yourself.

If you really don't want to eat things that are unhealthy for
you around the holidays, think of the candy as the damaging
force it really is. No matter how much we love it, sugar is
not good for us. Eating candy is like digging a hole. One bite
can be the first shovel-full of dirt. Do you really want to
risk falling into that hole?

Action for the day:

Treat yourself by putting those unhealthy foods out of sight
as best you can, and resolve to eat only satisfying, healthy
foods today.

Purge the junk food from your pantry.

Have you noticed that no matter how hard you try to keep junk food out of your house, somehow the bad stuff creeps back in? Once it's in the house, junk food is much harder to resist. And once you put that first bite in your body, the ability to resist the second and third is harder still.

Every once in awhile, go through your cupboards and get rid of the junk food that has accumulated. Your health and sanity are worth it.

Action for the day:

Vow to purge your cupboard of junk food today. If you feel resistant, ask a friend to come over and help you do it.

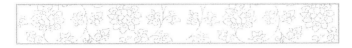

Fight alligators.

Think about all the fears and worries you have in your
day-to-day life—the alligators big and small you wrestle with.
Are many of them based on mistaken beliefs? Beliefs like,
"I can't maintain my weight loss," or "I am too fat to take
an exercise class."

Remember, fears and worries are not facts. The reality is you
can maintain your weight loss. The reality is you can
take an exercise class and no one will care about your size.
It's time to fight back all the imaginary alligators in your
life—the fears and worries that keep you too guarded and
missing out on fun.

Action for the day:

Do you spend your precious time fighting alligators? If so,
start fighting back. In your journal today, write a letter to
your fear-alligators and tell them you will not be needing
them anymore.

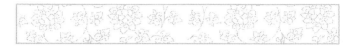

Don't let them wear you down.

Everyone, at some point in their lives, encounters a know-it-all. You may have someone like that in your life right now. Perhaps this person is convinced that she knows exactly what you should be eating and how frequently. You may have attempted to educate her about the reality of post-WLS life and why you make the decisions you make, and still she doesn't listen.

Some people are just not able to learn from others. So, don't argue. Interact with the know-it-all at about the same level you would with a shopping clerk. Be pleasant and talk about the weather—but don't let her steal your resolve.

Action for the day:

Is there someone in your life who constantly argues with you or criticizes you? If it's a friend, you may need to back off from the friendship to some degree. If it's a family member or coworker, and you cannot avoid her, change the subject or walk away whenever she tries to belittle or question your choices.

November

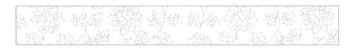

Eat three meals a day.

It's surprising how many weight loss surgery patients skip meals, thinking they are doing themselves a favor. But, skipping meals can actually lead to weight gain. (Did you know sumo wrestlers are told to skip breakfast to help them gain weight?)

Skipping a meal can also lead to excessive hunger and poor food choices later on, which leads to overeating.

Action for the day:

Eat three meals today, and have a protein-based snack if you are going to go more than five hours without food.

Think the bite through.

If you are a WLS patient who wants to avoid unhealthy snacking, change your focus and think the snack through. Before you take that first unhealthy bite, think about how it will create guilt and anxiety—how it will cause you to lose some of the self respect you've gained since having WLS. Consider how it will feel to lose your newfound freedom, your ability to move, the pleasure of having enough energy to be productive.

It's hard sometimes to make yourself think about the consequences of your actions, but if you are going to have long-term success you might want to start thinking the bite through.

Action for the day:

Today, if you find yourself reaching for an unhealthy bite, think it through. What will be the short- and long-term consequences?

Rejoice.

Have you taken the time to stop and think about how amazing weight loss surgery is? While most people would prefer to get healthy without having to go through surgery, at least there is a tool available that can bring great opportunity.

Take a moment to rejoice. Weight loss surgery is a gift, imperfect though it can be at times. And you can use WLS as a tool to help fulfill your dreams.

Action for the day:

Spend a quiet minute in reflection today. Rejoice that you have a tool to help you, and think about where you would be now without it. Are you using this gift to its full potential?

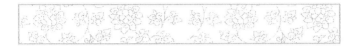

Get clear.

When you have clear expectations about how you want your post-WLS life to work, you will benefit greatly. Develop a detailed vision of how your life as a healthy person must look if you are to succeed. Who will you spend time with? What will you eat? How will you avoid unhealthy foods?

The people around you will be able to support you better if you are clear. For example, as the spouse or friend of a WLS patient, it's hard to be supportive if the patient eschews all desserts one day and brings home a bag of cookies the next.

Action for the day:

Do you have a clear vision of how your life needs to be established if you are to succeed at WLS? Spend some time today visualizing your ideal, healthy life. Write down your ideas in your journal.

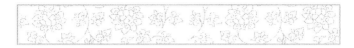

Have some absolutes.

The trouble with having an overeating problem is you can't swear off food completely. You have to eat. In addition, you are around all kinds of food all the time. It's hard to resist. While there are plenty of gray areas when it comes to the WLS lifestyle, you can have some absolutes.

To give yourself some freedom over uncertainty, consider selecting a few foods or behaviors to which you will apply absolute rules. Be absolute about not eating refined sweets and carbohydrates, for example. Or, never drink soda. Or, walk every day.

Action for the day:

Pick one thing you can be absolute about that will benefit your health. Write a contract with yourself (and be sure to sign it) stating what you will always (or never) do in support of your WLS goals.

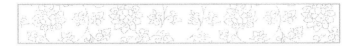

Attend to your spirit.

Your heart and soul need nurturing. Many people who have WLS are wounded souls. In fact, the same is probably true of the general population. Treating yourself kindly, listening to yourself, feeding your soul with love—these things are vital to how you will define yourself following WLS.

Take a gentle approach with yourself as you make time for attending to your spirit.

Action for the day:

Spend some time today being nurturing and loving toward yourself. Sometimes self nurturing takes a lot of practice. So, practice.

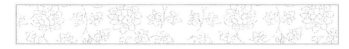

Motivate yourself to exercise.

It's not impossible to motivate yourself to exercise. Some people find motivation when they make a commitment to meet another person for a walk. Others get motivated when they are paying a personal trainer. The key is to know that you can create your own motivation.

Be creative! Getting a dog that has to be walked will also give you a furry friend to keep you company while you exercise. And taking a volunteer job that requires physical exertion, like Meals on Wheels, will help you stay fit while helping another human being, too.

Action for the day:

You can get motivated to move. Today, make plans to exercise with a friend or to help a neighbor. Motivation will follow such actions.

Eat dense protein first.

Soft foods can be comforting and tasty, but they are risky for WLS patients. For people whose WLS includes a small stoma through which food will pass into the intestines, the soft food goes through so easily that you may not feel full at times. Consequently, eating these soft foods may put you at risk for consuming more calories than you need.

Include dense protein with every meal. The dense proteins— beef, chicken, fish, etc.—will help you feel full and will stay with you longer. And be sure to avoid drinking beverages with your meals.

Action for the day:

Have you gotten into the habit of eating soft foods that don't stay with you long? Record what you eat today and evaluate your diet. Add dense proteins as needed.

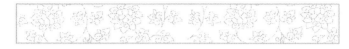

Be open-minded.

There is a saying: A closed system is a sick system. If you are
closed to new ideas, information, and support from others,
you are not nearly as likely to solve the problems that are
challenging you. When you do not seek out others for
support, your secrets and self-destructive behaviors will
discourage you and keep you down.

Open your mind to different people, approaches, and ideas,
or you will lose out on a great opportunity to find new
solutions and resources for long-term success.

Action for the day:

Take a moment today to explore your degree of open-
mindedness. Have you been open to trying new things to
help you succeed on your WLS journey?

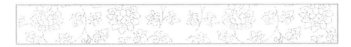

Make today count.

Sometimes life presents challenges that seem insurmountable. When tragedy strikes or plans fail, motivation can jump right out the window. When you're feeling discouraged, it's easy to lash out at others or mistreat yourself.

But have courage. Despite your circumstances, make today memorable for something positive. A positive action won't completely take your worries away, but it is the first step to overcoming adversity.

Action for the day:

No matter how you feel or what is happening in your life that is discouraging, take a positive action today. Make today count for something good.

Manage your mood.

When it comes to food, sometimes people let unchecked
emotions cloud their choices. When you are angry, you might
crave something crunchy. When you are sad, you might
want something warm and smooth. If you are an overeater,
you will most likely eat when your emotions are swelling.

Consider working on managing your mood. Many things can
affect your mood. You might have a chemical imbalance in
your brain. You might not be getting enough sleep. You might
have low blood sugar. You might be eating sweets. You might
be ignoring your real needs. Maybe you are unwilling to
feel certain feelings. No matter what the cause, allowing your
emotions to take over your life can lead to overeating.

Action for the day:

Are your moods ruling you? First of all, don't let yourself
get too hungry, angry, lonely, or tired. Second, meet with a
professional (for example, a therapist who specializes in food
addiction) to examine this aspect of your life and to determine
what you need to do to manage your mood in a healthy way.

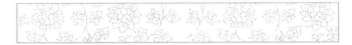

Push yourself.

Taking risks can be scary, but if you are not satisfied with some aspect of your life, then taking a risk just might be necessary to create change.

Getting out of your comfort zone may seem hard, but start small. If you practice taking risks, you will develop a tolerance. And once you are able to tolerate risk, you can take bold action to create a more satisfying life for yourself.

Action for the day:

Take a risk today—even a small one will do.

Consider switching to whole grains.

Instead of refined carbohydrates like white bread, pasta, and some cereals, consider consuming whole-grain products instead. (Your doctor or nutritionist should agree before you make any major changes in your diet.) Whole grains have important vitamins and minerals as well as fiber.

These days it's pretty easy to find whole-grain versions of your favorites. But, beware. Don't be fooled by the labels that say, "MADE WITH WHOLE GRAINS." These labels are misleading because the foods are unlikely to be made with only whole grains. These foods probably will have a significant amount of unrefined carbs in them, as well.

Action for the day:

Today, choose a food you eat often that is made with refined carbohydrates. Find a whole-grain substitute for that food and give it a try.

Be deliberate.

Think about what you are doing as you move through your day. It's easy to do the same things over and over again because you are used to a routine. But if that routine includes some self-defeating behaviors, it's time to make some different choices.

By deliberately choosing to create a healthier pattern to your life, you can gain some control over your eating and your life.

Action for the day:

If you normally stop in at a coffee shop on the way to work and order a muffin along with your latte, fix a healthy drink at home (a coffee-flavored protein shake, for example) and skip the coffee shop. Be deliberate in your choices today.

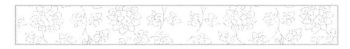

Renew your commitment to chew.

Do you inhale your food sometimes? After your surgery, it's easy to eat slowly, because if you don't you can get sick. Later on, eating fast gets easier, unfortunately. Part of a successful WLS program is to be willing to start over again, as often as necessary.

So, if you are back to eating too fast, start over. Make a conscious decision to eat your meals more slowly. Chew each bite at least 20 times, and put your fork down between bites. You will be more satisfied with less food.

Action for the day:

Instead of reading this and forgetting about it, make a commitment to yourself to eat one meal slowly today.

Choose foods wisely.

Long-term success is really a numbers game. You have to
expend more calories than you consume. To that end, make
wise food choices.

You don't have to sacrifice good taste and satisfaction for
good health. Just substitute tasty, healthy foods for tasty,
unhealthy foods. For example, instead of putting peanut
butter on crackers, spread peanut butter on celery sticks.
Choose the new high-fiber bread that has fewer calories per
slice than your regular whole grain bread. Or, eat fresh, ripe
pineapple instead of a handful of gummy bears.

Action for the day:

Write down a food plan just for today. Review it and
brainstorm to see if you can make some healthy substitutions
that won't sacrifice your satisfaction.

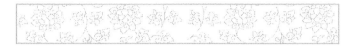

Recharge your batteries.

You don't have to adopt a Scrooge-like attitude toward the coming holiday season. Despite all of the commercialism and the intense, unhealthy focus on food and drink, the holidays can be a time of joy and contentment. But even the most optimistic, upbeat person needs a break from the excitement to recharge.

The intense holiday season lasts more than a month nowadays, and you'll start seeing evidence of it soon (if you haven't already). When you find yourself caught up in the excitement, remember to step back once in awhile to take a breather. It will reenergize you, help you avoid the burnout that could lead to stress eating, and provide you with the boost you need to stay on track.

Action for the day:

Today, before the upcoming holidays begin to consume you, write down a plan for how you will handle the coming season. With a plan, you are much more likely to stay on track.

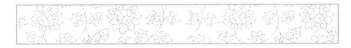

Choose realistic goals.

When setting goals, it's okay to start small. Pick realistic goals, and get used to the feeling of achieving them. For example, if you haven't been exercising, set a timer and walk for 10 minutes around your living room every day for a week. Then add three minutes to your walks each week, eventually moving your walks outdoors.

There will be plenty of time down the road to set higher goals. Start small, and build a successful record from which you can draw courage and strength.

Action for the day:

Choose one realistic goal today, and take a small action to move toward it.

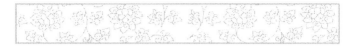

Do weight training.

One tool that is awesome for weight loss and maintenance is weight training. Resistance and weightlifting exercises will help keep your metabolism humming. You'll be burning more calories. And you don't necessarily have to join a gym to do them; you can perform many of these exercises just about anywhere.

If you are inexperienced with weight training, it is worth the expense to hire a personal trainer to develop a weight-training program for you. And be sure to check with your doctor before beginning any exercise program.

Action for the day:

Research weight training and come up with a plan of action to add this tool to your WLS toolkit.

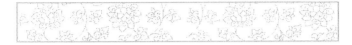

Reframe your problems.

Looking at your problems as opportunities is a way to practice a "can-do" attitude. It's a concrete way to begin to change the way you think. And it's a great way to get out of self pity.

You can turn a problem into an opportunity by using a simple statement: I used to have trouble with (state the problem), but now I choose to (state the solution). For example, say, "I used to arrive home too hungry and binge on crackers when I came home from work, but now I eat an apple and a cheese stick at my desk before I leave work."

Action for the day:

Make a list of your problems, making sure to feel all the self pity and woe you can muster. Then reframe them by writing them out in your journal, as demonstrated above.

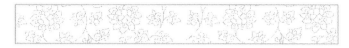

Be someone's life preserver.

Most WLS patients know what they should be doing to be successful. But almost everyone struggles from time to time. When you are struggling, do you find it hard to reach out for help? A lot of people feel so bad about what they are doing, they retreat in shame.

So, if you are in a good place, reach out to someone who may be struggling. You don't need to judge them. Just let them know you understand, and that you're there for them. Remind them they are worthy.

Action for the day:

Think about someone who you know is struggling with maintaining their WLS lifestyle. Give them a call today and offer your support.

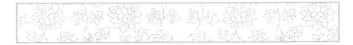

Let feelings be feelings and facts be facts.

One of the biggest mistakes human beings can make is to base certain lifestyle decisions on feelings. When you are in the process of changing to a healthier lifestyle, you will feel uncomfortable with the change, so you may make decisions to do certain things based on your feelings—like drinking with your meals because you enjoy the flavor of the beverage.

When creating a healthier lifestyle, it is wiser to base your decisions on facts. Exercise, for example, is critical to long-term success. So, not feeling like exercising is irrelevant. You have to look at the bigger questions: What are my long-term goals and what will get me there? The factual answers to those questions should be what you base your decisions on.

Action for the day:

Do something you don't feel like doing today, because you know it will make you healthier (and happier in the long run).

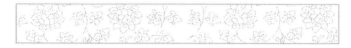

Live and let live.

It's easy to confuse someone else's unhappiness for your own.
But, taking on another's pain can harm you. You can show
compassion to others, but let them live their own lives and
feel their own feelings. That is how they will grow as human
beings.

It's your job to live your life, and feel your own feelings. That
is how you will grow as a human being. Neglecting yourself
will not help others in the long run.

Action for the day:

Are you allowing someone else's problems or feelings to get in
the way of your sense of well being? Today, when you begin
to feel too much for others, send a heart-felt prayer up for
them, and then return your focus to your own critical needs.

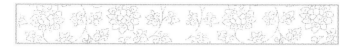

Be yourself.

How many of us spend hours, days, weeks, months, even years, doing what we think others want us to do, rather than what we want to do?

What in this world is exciting to you? What will make your heart sing? Maybe you cannot put down what you are doing right now and pick up an exciting new challenge. But, you can start to plan, do some research, and begin to visualize the satisfied and fully authentic you.

Action for the day:

In your journal, write down a list of things that really excite you.

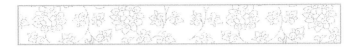

Consider joining a gym or taking a class.

Have you been avoiding the gym or exercise classes because you think you need to be fit first? This attitude can be self defeating. Why not jump start your fitness process (and it is a process) by trying something new? Sometimes having a dedicated place to work out, or being committed to a class, is motivating. You can try out different equipment (this is very helpful if it's been a long time since you've exercised) and discover new types of movement you enjoy.

If you are worried about feeling too awkward, hire a personal trainer to work out with you for the first few weeks until you get more comfortable. Or, recruit a WLS friend to join the gym or class with you.

Action for the day:

If you haven't done so already, choose three gyms in your area and make plans to tour them. You don't have to join when you take a tour. In fact, let them know you are visiting several facilities before you make a decision. If you find a gym you like, ask for a free pass to try it out before you actually join.

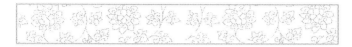

Accept compliments.

It sounds simple enough, doesn't it? If someone offers you a
compliment, you should accept it. But chances are you've
often felt tempted to dismiss the compliment—"Oh, don't
be silly, I didn't do anything special." Or, "You're kidding,
I look awful."

But dismissing those compliments is the same as dismissing
yourself. You're sending yourself—and the rest of the world—
a subtle message that you don't think you're worthy of praise.
But you are. So rejoice when you hear people complimenting
you. They really mean it and you really deserve it.

Action for the day:

When someone offers you a compliment, smile graciously
and say, "Thank you."

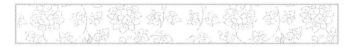

Seek support during the holidays.

It's the most wonderful time of the year…or so some people think. For many people, though, the holiday season is stressful and/or depressing. This is the time of year to seek support and give it. If you respond to stress with self-destructive behaviors (overcommitting, overeating, having unrealistic expectations of what you can handle) your holiday season will hinder your progress.

You don't have to surrender your sanity to the season. You don't have to bake. You don't have to eat the hors d'oeuvres. You don't have to spend more money than you have. Seek support for your new lifestyle if you need it. And offer to help others get through the holidays, too. Sometimes the best way to stay on track is by being an example to others who are struggling.

Action for the day:

Plan a realistic day today. Don't buy into the myth of having to do what everyone else is doing. And touch base with another WLS patient today to get and give support.

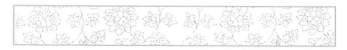

Continue to practice an attitude of gratitude.

With WLS, you have a new lease on life. You can eat less and still enjoy the flavor of food. You can take small bites and savor them—small bites of food and small bites of life.

Some WLS patients feel sorry for themselves on eating holidays. Don't give in to the temptation to feel sorry for yourself. Instead, tell yourself you are healing, strong, and hopeful. You have chosen a new life that will bring great rewards. Today you can focus on your new hope and patiently wait for the rewards to come.

Action for today:

In your journal, make a gratitude list. Save it so that next year at Thanksgiving time you can make a new one and compare the two. The rewards of your new life will be evident.

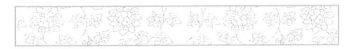

Understand your needs are important.

Life is demanding. It's easy to fill your days caring for others. But, now that you have had weight loss surgery, you must make time for your needs, too.

In fact, it's okay to put your needs first. Sure, on rare occasion someone needs something vital from you, but day to day, most of the things we put before our own needs are a choice. Try to develop the skills you need to resist putting others' needs first all the time. You deserve to be healthy and balanced—and your WLS success depends on it.

Action for the day:

Think about what you need to do for yourself today, and write those things down on your calendar. Fill in the needs of others around what you will be doing for yourself.

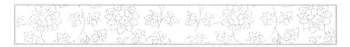

Be honest with yourself.

So, how did you do on Thanksgiving? Was it as hard as you feared? Was it easier than you thought it'd be? What was it like to watch others eat favorites you chose to pass up? Did you enjoy cooking for others, or did cooking trigger unpleasant food cravings for you?

Develop a battle plan for future holidays, based on how you handled the recent holiday. WLS recovery is a process of trial and error. None of us is perfect. We are works in progress. Our best hope for long-term weight loss maintenance is rigorous honesty. It really doesn't matter how you handled Thanksgiving, as long as you have learned from it.

Action for the day:

Make an honest list of what worked and what didn't work with regard to how you handled Thanksgiving. Next to what didn't work, write down a new plan of action for the next time you are in a similar situation. Review this list before your next holiday event.

December

Change your pace.

When you get bored with your routine, you are vulnerable to breaking it. Better to build in some variety than to go looking for it in a vulnerable moment.

You can change all sorts of things to keep life interesting. For example, if you walk at a fast pace when you're exercising, take a stroll instead and focus on your breath—breathe in for four paces and breathe out for four paces. If you normally take leisurely walks, pick up the pace. See if you can cover your usual distance in a shorter amount of time.

Action for the day:

Change something today to make your regimen more interesting. Do a different exercise, try a new spice, have a picnic for lunch, or eat dinner for breakfast—whatever sounds fun to you.

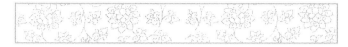

Give yourself a break.

Have you been hard on yourself lately? Do you criticize yourself at every misstep?

Negative self talk does not help you to change the behaviors you want to change. It is discouraging, and often leads to self-destructive behavior. So, instead of telling yourself you are fat, for example, tell yourself you are making progress, or that you are capable of change, or that you are lovable.

Action for the day:

Today, be nice to yourself. Talk kindly. Don't judge. Be encouraging. You may be surprised at how you respond to a break from the harshness.

Appreciate the little miracles.

Sometimes things go exactly right. You are in a hurry and all the traffic lights are green. You are making a recipe and you find that one, obscure ingredient in the back of your spice cabinet. You give someone a gift, and it turns out it's exactly what they wanted.

Life can be quite joyful when things go just right. From time to time, as sure as the sun comes up, things will go your way.

Action for the day:

Focus on what goes right today and appreciate the small miracles around you.

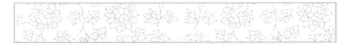

Enjoy the roller coaster.

Some people think they would be happier if life was without problems or challenges. But, the challenges make life interesting and exciting. Like a roller coaster, an exciting life is full of ups and downs, dread, anticipation, sharp turns, screams, and squeals of joy.

It's the merry-go-round that stays the same, always predictable. But it's just not as exciting. Sure, it has no real lows, no plunges into despair, but it also has no real highs, no moments that almost reach the stars.

Action for the day:

Be thankful today for the roller coaster ride of life. Appreciate the highs for the joy they provide and the lows for helping you understand what real joy is.

Identify where your feelings are.

When trying to master emotional eating, it is useful to identify where in your body you are feeling a feeling. You can ask yourself: What am I feeling? Where do I feel it? In my stomach? In my chest? In my legs? Then, ask yourself: Does this feeling make me want to eat? If so, what food comes to mind?

This is a simple exercise aimed at helping you develop awareness about your emotions and your food thoughts.

Action for the day:

Several times today, take a moment to check in with yourself. Try to sort out what you are feeling, where in your body you are feeling it, and what—if any—food thoughts you are having in response to your feelings.

Have a plan for holiday gatherings.

Holiday eating can be a source of stress after surgery. But, you can still enjoy the holiday and much of the food. Just make a plan. Everyone has certain strategies that work for them. Keep in mind what works for you as you make your plan.

One strategy is to take a tablespoon (or smaller if you have a tiny pouch) of anything you want to taste. Use a small spoon, like the disposable plastic baby spoons you can get at the grocery store, and a small plate, too. Eat your food slowly and pause between bites, so that you get maximum satisfaction from the food.

Action for the day:

Brainstorm and write down a list of strategies you will try this holiday season to keep you on track.

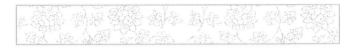

Mind your own business.

Just because you are in a relationship with someone—just because you love someone—doesn't mean you have to join with them in their unhealthy thinking and behavior. Nor are you responsible for their actions. It's not your job to fix them or solve the problems that arise as a result of their negative actions and feelings.

Your responsibility is to live your own life, not to obsess about someone else's problems. It's okay to take care of yourself even when those around you are struggling.

Action for the day:

Today focus on your own business instead of someone else's. Give yourself the much-needed love and attention you deserve.

Live in the gray area.

Are you plagued by an "all or nothing" attitude? Do you find it hard to make healthy choices when you have made one tiny misstep?

It's time to get comfortable with the gray areas in life. It's time to allow yourself progress, even if you are not perfect. It is better to move forward three steps and back one than it is not to move forward at all.

Action for the day:

Be gentle with yourself today and allow yourself to make imperfect progress.

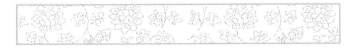

Redefine exercise.

Do you balk when you hear the word exercise?

You don't have to "exercise" if you hate exercise. You can mow the lawn, do home improvement projects, walk the dog, make pottery, or even play twister with your kids. Some people carry in their own groceries and weed their own gardens. Some people dance in the living room when no one else is home. Do whatever works for you, but don't pass up this great tool.

Action for the day:

Do something to move your body today. Be as creative as you need to be to make it interesting and palatable.

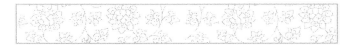

Role play.

Changing your behaviors and actions can be a daunting task.
And when your change requires you to set new boundaries
with people, you may find yourself putting off a boundary-
setting talk you need to have with someone.

Practicing what you want to say and how you want to say it
will make those boundary-setting conversations much easier.
You can write out what points you need to cover, practice
with a safe friend what you will say and do, and only then
carry out the real conversation.

Action for the day:

Select one person with whom you need to set a new bound-
ary. In your journal, write down what you want to say, then
do a role play with a friend. Finally, have the conversation!

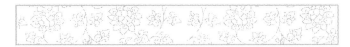

Get your game face on.

The holiday season is heating up now. People are having parties, going caroling, shopping, and baking like crazy.

Put on your game face now. It's time to get serious about your goals and your needs. Rather than use the holidays as an excuse to throw caution to the wind, use them to improve your health-building skills. Winning means you practice hard, take your lumps, and make real progress. It is an attitude and a way of life. Your challenge has been laid out. Are you ready to rumble?

Action for the day:

Get a notebook and label it, "WLS Game Plan for the Holidays." Write down a list of the games you will be facing: family gatherings, office parties, gifts of baked goods, etc. Under each item, make a list of strategies you can use to be a winner.

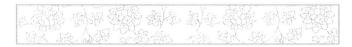

Look for beauty.

An empty field can be many things to many people. To a
developer it's a potential financial windfall in the form of a
new shopping center; to an environmentalist it's a habitat for
an endangered species; to a child it's a field of dreams. The
bottom line, though, is that it's always the same field no
matter who is looking at it. Many of the daily choices you
make—and the attitudes you hold—are more reflections of
yourself than anything else.

You can see beauty in many things or you can see ugliness.
Try to be aware of your biases creeping in as you view
yourself and your life. The more willing you are to see beauty
in you and the world around you, the more positive your
daily choices will be.

Action for the day:

Spend some time today meditating on the beauty in you
and around you. Challenge yourself to focus on the beauty
you realize.

Avoid comparing your insides to their outsides.

The problem with comparing yourself to others is that it's always a case of comparing apples and oranges. Even if you personally know the person you're measuring yourself against, it can never be an accurate comparison. Nobody completely knows another person.

Perhaps that successful person at work is struggling in her home life. Perhaps your neighbor with the immaculate yard struggles with a secret addiction. The only person you should compare yourself to is you. As you continue to change, compare the old you to the new you. See how far you've come, and what you still need to work on.

Action for the day:

Today, try to avoid comparing yourself to others. Measure yourself against the old you, and congratulate yourself on how far you've come.

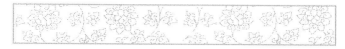

Put off the next bite.

If you are having a day in which you are thinking about food nonstop, you can adopt some strategies to get you through for the short run, and start a process to overcome your grazing or emotional eating in the long run.

To stop the grazing in the short run, try putting off your eating. One strategy is to set a timer to go off when you can have your next meal, and keep yourself busy until you hear the bell. Another is to start a task that will take up all your time until your next meal. Tell yourself you'll eat when you've gotten all your papers filed, for example.

Action for the day:

If you have the urge to graze today, put it off by using a new strategy. Then, in your journal, write about how you were feeling when you began to crave the food, and how it felt to use your new strategy instead of eating.

Draw a line in the sand.

With weight regain being so common, it is helpful to set up some parameters for yourself, so that you know how you're going to handle it when the scale creeps up.

Choose a weight beyond which you do not want to gain. When you get close to that weight, implement a plan to take care of the extra weight right away. Waiting will only invite more regain. So, know your line in the sand and vow not to cross it.

Action for the day:

Do you know where your line in the sand is? Choose it today. And write in your journal the plan you will follow if you get close to your line.

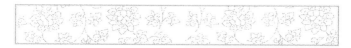

Define yourself.

The people who know you best have come to expect certain things from you—some positive and some negative. They may know, for example, that historically when you have gotten stressed at work you've come home with a take-out pizza and a soda.

After WLS, you will need to redefine yourself in others' eyes. You will need to teach them who the new you is and what the new you does. Clear communication will be important, as will be consistency.

Action for the day:

Redefine yourself. In your journal, write down, "Now that I have had WLS, I am different. Now, I...." Then, complete that thought.

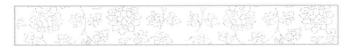

Affirm yourself.

You've heard of positive affirmations, no doubt. Do you think it's just another bit of psychobabble? Or, a flaky part of the new-age movement? If you have those thoughts, think again. Positive affirmations are statements about your better self. They describe the part of you who wanted to lose weight and be healthy, finally—and for good.

Your mind probably plays old tapes—familiar self-defeating thoughts like, "The other shoe is going to drop eventually. It always does," and, "I can't control my grazing." Positive affirmations are one way of erasing the old tapes. So give it a try. Unless you want to listen to the old tapes. Do you?

Action for the day:

In your journal, write down an affirmation that refutes an old tape that has been influencing you lately. Write the affirmation down on a card to carry with you, and resolve to say it every time you notice that old tape playing in your mind.

Visualize.

To change a behavior that has become a well-worn path in your life, you must do the work of creating a new path. You will need to remove brush, flatten the ground, and maybe even do some paving to make your new path smooth.

It's not all physical labor, though. Change in behavior involves a mental component. Each time you visualize yourself taking the new path or behaving in a new way, you are creating your new path. Simply by sitting quietly and visualizing, you create change.

Action for the day:

Today, take a few minutes to visualize the healthy behavior you want to adopt.

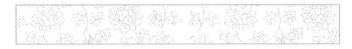

Meditate.

Is your life so busy you have trouble taking time for yourself?
Do you have a tough time finding quiet moments for
introspection? Being too busy to focus on your needs and
your spirit is a more serious problem than you may think.
It's a subtle form of self sabotage.

Meditating is an easy way to take time for yourself, and it is
an activity from which you can reap great rewards. Even
investing a small amount of time will help tremendously.
There are numerous books written about meditation. Research
the subject if you wish, or you may choose to just keep it
simple. Try sitting quietly, closing your eyes, and breathing
deeply—four counts in and four counts out. In and out.

Action for the day:

Find a quiet place and meditate for five minutes today.

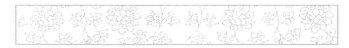

Give yourself permission to have fun.

Feeling stressed or depressed about the holidays? Give yourself permission to lighten up and have some fun. Feelings of frustration, stress, loneliness, gloominess, or discouragement are not permanent conditions. All feelings pass.

Why not willfully put aside some of your woes today and look at the lighter side of life? Find something to laugh about. Play. Watch an old movie you love. Remember, life is too short to be serious all the time.

Action for the day:

Right now, write yourself a permission slip to play. Decorate it and post it in a visible place. Then, use it.

Assess your mental condition.

Your mind needs to adjust to the major changes you've gone through. You have behavior patterns to correct, emotions to process, and information to learn. But where do you begin?

Assess your mental condition and address your issues in that arena. For example, if you are feeling depressed, go talk to a professional about it. If you are confused about what you are supposed to be doing regarding your WLS, seek out experts who can provide you with good information. If you want to change your habits, get support and information so that you can work on the changes you want to make in a more productive way.

Action for the day:

Think about your mind today. Are you doing what you need to do to make a mentally healthy adjustment to the new you? If not, begin today.

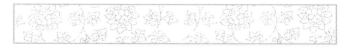

Tell yourself this too shall pass.

If the holidays have put a dent in your healthy lifestyle, it's time to forgive yourself and know the holidays will end shortly. You will soon be moving on and getting back into your healthier habits.

When you are in a bad place with food, the fear is that you will be there forever. But you won't be. This too shall pass. Tell yourself that and start making plans for better days. They are just around the corner.

Action for the day:

In your journal, write a loving and healthy plan for tomorrow that will help you feel in control of your eating and your life.

Pare down your to-do list.

If you find that your to-do list is longer than a child's jump rope, you may need to downsize your obligations. Is everything on your list really necessary? Or could some things be eliminated?

Do you really need that third car, for example, given the amount of time you have to devote to its maintenance? Would your children (and you) be happier if you eliminated field hockey practice and limited your children to one sport each quarter? You're likely to find that whittling down your to-do list is an instant stress reliever.

Action for the day:

Study your to-do list. (Write it down if you keep it all in your head.) Then, pick at least one thing to eliminate. And if you can get yourself to do it, eliminate three things.

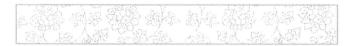

Remember what is important.

In the final days of rushing around before the holiday, it's easy to get crazy. Not only do you want to make everything special for your family, you also want to do things for your friends. You may feel obligated to do things for other people in your life as well, like your child's teachers or a business partner.

This is the time to ask: What really matters? If you could reflect on your life the way Scrooge was able to do in *A Christmas Carol*, what would you want to see happening?

Action for the day:

The holidays can be a crazy time. Focus on what really matters today.

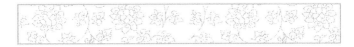

Keep your power.

When you let someone else's needs and desires determine
your agenda, you are giving away your power—and you
potentially are creating a feeling of helplessness in yourself.

To make long-term health gains, you need to feel and be
empowered. No one can look out for your health and your
needs the way you can. When you allow someone to binge
on cookies in front of you or to insist you watch a TV show
with them instead of going on your walk, you are giving
away your power.

Action for the day:

Today, consider whether your choices are based on pleasing
someone else or on your own health needs. If you've been
giving your power away, reclaim it.

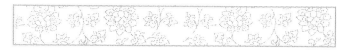

Finish the year on an up note.

You've made it through most of the holidays now. You've made some good choices and maybe some not-so-good choices. New Year's Eve will be here soon. Use the tips and tricks you've learned along the way to finish your year on an up note.

If you're going to a party, bring a WLS-friendly dish to share. Make a point to take small bites and chew thoroughly. Use a smaller plate. If it's a buffet, let someone you trust put food on your plate and bring it to you. Don't drink with your meals. Plan things to do with your hands other than eating: knitting, puzzles, games. Don't skip one meal in anticipation of the next. Remember, small choices matter.

Action for the day:

Make a plan for the remainder of your holiday season. What a great way to kick off your new year.

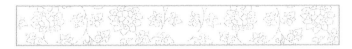

Skip the alcohol.

It may be tradition to drink alcohol on New Year's Eve, but alcohol can be risky for WLS patients, depending on your type of surgery. For example, people who have had gastric bypass may become more easily intoxicated than before their surgery.

But did you know that alcohol has 7 calories per gram, while protein and veggies have 4 calories per gram? That is why people who start drinking again after surgery can have more trouble losing weight or more easily gain weight. More importantly, though, alcohol can become an addiction for those already struggling with food.

Action for the day:

Think about how your behavior with alcohol can affect your WLS recovery. Maybe it's worth skipping. And if you suspect you may have a problem with alcohol, please seek help.

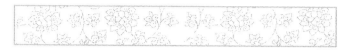

Reflect first, then plan.

On New Year's Eve, many people talk about their plans for the coming year. They make resolutions and hope for better times ahead. But before you start down the resolution path, pause for a moment and truly reflect. What can you learn from the past year about yourself? Have you discovered what works in terms of your health and what doesn't?

You can make resolutions soon (or better yet, set goals), but today look back. You owe it to yourself to learn your lessons, so that you can grow wiser and healthier in the coming year.

Action for the day:

Even if you usually don't journal, take a few minutes to do this exercise. Make a list of things you wish you had done differently this past year, and then a list of what you did well. Next to the things you wish you had done differently, write down a step you can take to ensure you won't repeat that mistake. Next to the things you did well write down what you can do to continue having success in that area. Read this list every morning in January.

Refocus on your needs.

Have you been so busy you forgot to take care of yourself? If so, it's time to regroup.

The longer you live the WLS lifestyle, the less urgent it seems to make healthy choices. But when you disregard your own needs, even to care for others, you do yourself—and them—a disservice. Today, remind yourself that your WLS lifestyle is effective only when you stop and acknowledge you have the disease of obesity, and that you need to be treating it whether you are overweight or not.

Action for the day:

Take a few minutes today to plan what you will do to refocus on your health needs in the coming year. Write down your plans and refer to them often.

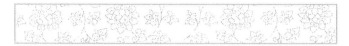

Get enough sleep.

Do you put off going to bed so that you can have quiet time for yourself, even though you have to get up early? Do you place a higher value on a lot of things besides sleep?

Insufficient sleep is tied to weight regain. It's harder to follow a healthy food plan when you're tired. In fact, everything is much more difficult when you're tired. Lack of sleep is one of the biggest problems people have, and the most underestimated in its impact on your health.

Action for the day:

Start a log to find out how much sleep you're really getting. Find a way to get more rest, if needed.

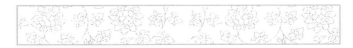

Try, try again.

Sometimes after the holidays it's hard to get back on track again. Maybe you've put on a few pounds and feel huge. Maybe you feel like you cannot control your eating. Please know this feeling will pass.

Keep trying. Start over every minute if you have to. And eat dense protein. Even if you have to bake chicken for breakfast, do it. Make tasty, "safe" foods, such as stewed chicken and vegetables. Eat good foods you like at every meal until you start to feel more satisfied and in control. It's hard to feel yucky when you eat solid, healthy food.

Action for the day:

Get back to basics. Eat dense protein and well-prepared, nutrient-rich vegetables at every meal today.

Acknowledgments

Small Bites has been a labor of love on the part of many individuals. A special thank you to Julia Persing, my friend, walking buddy, fellow dreamer, and co-author. Other writers and editors contributed bits and pieces to this book, including Mariane Mears, Alyssa Joy, Kathy Steam, Natalie J. Damschroder, Cathy Wilson, and Carole Campbell. Emily Peace contributed a beautiful book design, and offered support and encouragement along the way. Many thanks to you all. Finally, I want to acknowledge and thank the readers of the *Small Bites* newsletter and the members of the National Association for Weight Loss Surgery for their support, encouragement, and enthusiasm for this project.

Katie Jay

Index

S

self acceptance, see acceptance, of self

self assertion, 78, 199, 206, 280

self awareness, 39, 62, 65, 75, 86, 181, 205, 216, 227, 268, 271, 311, 343, 368
    and intuition, 121

self control, 54, 100
    as perfectionism, 296, 359

self-destructive behavior, 32, 74, 84, 295
    and remembering the past, 53

self discipline, 123, 180, 236, 273, 299, 333

self esteem, 54, 65, 144, 250

self image, 29, 76, 103
    and perception, 46, 58, 67, 363

self respect, 103, 282, 321

self sacrifice, 142

self worth, 104, 144, 364, 376

skin, excess, 31

sleep, 262, 381

staying in the present, 6, 49, 66, 88,147, 176, 194, 261, 284, 329

stomach, smaller, 10

stress, 4, 99, 107, 149, 186, 266, 275
    and resentment, 22
    slowing down to relieve, 178
    related to clutter, 253

success
    acceptance of, 8
    and making a schedule, 14
    and too many responsibilities, 47, 264, 305, 374
    small changes to reaching, 64
    by "faking it till you make it," 101
    through redefining yourself, 110
    plan for rebellion to reach, 145
    when old habits return, 164
    living with guilt and, 169
    and humility, 172
    by learning from mistakes, 217

sugar
    abstinence from, 166

About the authors

Katie Jay, MSW, is director of the National Association for Weight Loss Surgery (www.nawls.com), a certified life coach, and author of *Dying to Change: My Really Heavy Life Story, How Weight Loss Surgery Gave Me Hope for Living*. Her passion is to help people find long-term success after WLS. Katie has been addressing issues such as addiction, eating disorders, and cognitive and behavioral lifestyle changes for more than 20 years.

As a successful WLS recipient, Katie is a leading spokesperson for WLS. She has been interviewed on CNN Radio and has also been featured in *The National Enquirer* and *Woman's World*.

Katie earned her Masters in Social Work from Virginia Commonwealth University and her undergraduate degree in Writing from George Mason University (GMU).

She draws on years of corporate experience from her "first career" as a communications manager, business writer, and editor. She lives in North Carolina (near the beach) with her husband Mike, son Barrett, and their delightfully annoying animal friends Lucy and Ruby.

Julia A. F. Persing resides in North Carolina with her husband and four children. Julia has led a life of struggle with her weight. She struggled with anorexia in college and obesity most of her adult life, seeking help continually. She graduated with a degree in biology from the University of Cincinnati, where she met her beloved husband. After marrying, she took graduate courses and taught high school science. With the birth of her first child, she became an at-home mom. Four children later she met Katie Jay, who had undergone WLS, changing her own life, and subsequently Julia's.

Katie Jay coaches weight loss surgery patients who understand that WLS is not a magic cure

Says Katie, "Many of my coaching clients come to me hoping to make more progress in their lives: with their WLS goals, in their relationships, at work, and in other areas. They have certain challenges that are hard to overcome—like a spouse who isn't supporting their WLS lifestyle, an unyielding desire to graze on refined carbs, or a special-needs child who zaps the time the client needs to take care of him or herself.

Other clients just feel lost. They've had their surgery and they are losing weight (sometimes not as much as they'd like), but they don't know what else they need to be doing. And they are worried about their future.

A coach is often the one person in your life whose only goal is to support you in your goal-setting, growth, and fulfillment. Coaches establish a partnership with you and together we create strategies and action plans that move you forward in your life—which brings you the results you've been longing for."

"Katie, thank you for being there and helping me remember the goals I made for myself before I had WLS and how to better use this wonderful tool…to become a much more healthy person." —Julie B., NAWLS Member

You can email Katie for more information at katiejay@nawls.com.

Katie Jay speaks to groups and organizations about obesity sensitivity and weight loss surgery

In her book, *Dying to Change: My Really Heavy Life Story, How Weight Loss Surgery Gave Me Hope for Living*, Katie Jay chronicles the life and challenges of a food addict and obesity survivor.

Katie's unique perspective, along with her mental health background, makes her an ideal speaker for groups and organizations who require obesity sensitivity training.

In addition to her talk, Katie gives each sensitivity-training participant a copy of her book. It's Katie's way of helping bring compassion and respect to those who still suffer with obesity.

You can email Katie for more information at katiejay@nawls.com.

Katie Jay leads workshops

If you are enjoying this book and would like to learn more about how to be successful with weight loss surgery and life, consider one of Katie Jay's intensive WLS Advantage™ workshops.

For about the same cost as a trip to the grocery store, you can benefit from a full-day of Katie's top-notch advice and guidance. And you'll appreciate the opportunity to explore your WLS journey and challenge your old ideas in a nonjudgmental setting. Katie's workshops are $195—and will help you make the most of the surgery that cost you $25,000+. (Also, they're great fun!)

You'll get insight, strategies, and practical tips on creating a healthy and balanced life; maintaining your weight loss; and finding peace with your body, mind, and spirit. This is not a diet and calories meeting. It's information and discussion about how to change your thinking and behavior so you can be successful after surgery.

Workshops are available by request. Just find 10 friends who want to know the truth about how to make WLS work for them and contact Katie with your request. She'd be happy to conduct a workshop in your city, schedule allowing.

You can email Katie for more information at katiejay@nawls.com.

Notes:

Notes:

Notes: